Language Sampling with Adolescents

Implications for Intervention

Second Edition

D0878836

Language Sampling with Adolescents

Implications for Intervention

Second Edition

Marilyn A. Nippold, PhD, CCC-SLP

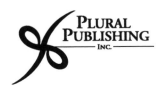

PLURAL
PUBLISHING
INC.

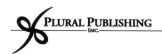

5521 Ruffin Road
San Diego, CA 92123

e-mail: info@pluralpublishing.com
Website: http://www.pluralpublishing.com

Typeset in 11/13 Garamond by Flanagan's Publishing Services, Inc.
Printed in the United States of America by McNaughton & Gunn, Inc.
20 19 18 17   3 4 5 6

Library of Congress Cataloging-in-Publication Data

Nippold, Marilyn A., 1951- author.
 Language sampling with adolescents : implications for intervention / Marilyn A.
Nippold.—Second edition.
    p. ; cm.
 Includes bibliographical references and index.
 ISBN 978-1-59756-570-7 (alk. paper)—ISBN 1-59756-570-9 (alk. paper)
 I. Title.
 [DNLM: 1. Language Disorders—diagnosis. 2. Language Tests. 3. Adolescent.
4. Language Development. 5. Language Disorders—therapy. 6. Speech-Language
Pathology—methods. WL 340.2]
 RJ496.S7
 618.92'85506—dc23
            2014000155

Contents

Preface

*I*n June 1972, I graduated from the University of California Los Angeles with a B.A. degree in philosophy, also having studied psychology. That autumn, instead of reading the works of Plato and Piaget, I began working as a teacher's assistant in a preschool program for low-income families in Southern California. Whenever the speech-language pathologist came into the classroom to evaluate the children who spoke very little or whose speech was unclear or disfluent, I observed with great interest as I continued my duties of setting up for snack, cleaning paint brushes, organizing bookshelves, and creating seasonal bulletin boards. By the end of the school year, having had the opportunity to observe individual and small-group therapy sessions, I knew that I had found my calling—to become a speech-language pathologist and work with children.

Thus, I spent the summer of 1973 taking classes in communicative disorders at nearby California State University Long Beach where I read the works of scholars such as Roger Brown (1973), Noam Chomsky (1965), Mildred Berry (1969), and Mildred Templin (1957). Upon learning about the concept of spontaneous language sampling, I began audio-recording conversations with neighborhood children as they happily talked about story books, pets, and favorite activities. I then transcribed their samples by hand, laboriously calculating mean length of utterance (MLU) in words, and attempting to analyze their speech with an emerging program called *Developmental Sentence Scoring*, or DSS (Lee & Canter, 1971). After that summer, I entered the master's degree program at California State University Long Beach, confident in my choice of career and eager to learn more about it.

After earning my M.A. degree in 1976, I began working as a speech-language pathologist in Southern California, first in a private clinic with preschool children, and later in a public school with young adolescents. During those years, I continued to learn about language development and disorders, reading books and articles and attending conferences. I also continued to record, transcribe, and analyze my clients' conversations. At the time, it was easy to find information on how to analyze the spoken language of young children. However, I was hard pressed to find solid guidance from textbooks, journals, or conferences that would help me to evaluate the spoken language of children over the age of 7 years. Although it was obvious to me that language development continued well beyond that point, little research had been published on later language development or on language disorders in school-age children and adolescents.

My work as a speech-language pathologist with adolescents was particularly heartbreaking. For those young people, the years of struggling with a language disorder had impacted them greatly, gradually eroding their self-esteem, social development, and school success. Unfortunately, none of my students could read or write at grade level or speak with clarity, precision, or confidence. However, I believed that much could be done to help them succeed, if more information were available from research on later language development.

In the spring of 1978, I was accepted into the doctoral program in speech-language pathology at Purdue University in West Lafayette, Indiana. As a doctoral student, my goal was to learn as much as possible about language development and language disorders in school-age children and adolescents. Since graduating from Purdue in 1982, I have been on the faculty in Communication Disorders and Sciences at the University of Oregon, where I have continued to learn about later language development and disorders, by conducting research projects in areas such as figurative language understanding, word learning, metalinguistics, verbal reasoning, reading, and spoken and written discourse.

This book on language sampling with adolescents is an effort to pull together some of my recent projects on discourse development, in an applied format. Its major purpose is to provide guidance for eliciting, transcribing, and analyzing conversational, narrative, expository, and persuasive discourse samples with students in grades 5 through 12 (ages 10–18 years). Suggestions are offered on how to use that information to promote students' language development. The book is written for speech-language pathologists who struggle, as I have, to make intervention relevant and effective for older students.

Speech-language pathologists who work in the schools often are called upon to evaluate the spoken and written language skills of adolescents, an activity that should include language sampling in order to learn how well young people communicate in natural settings. This information then can be used to design intervention activities to assist students in meeting Common Core State Standards and in helping them to excel at formal speaking and writing assignments in the classroom. Speech-language pathologists are ideally suited for conducting these activities because of the extensive training they receive in language development and disorders. However, language sampling with adolescents can be challenging. For example, speech-language pathologists often report that they are unfamiliar with language sampling tasks that are appropriate for adolescents; that they are unsure of how to encourage adolescents to talk; and that they have little understanding of how to analyze a sample, not knowing what to expect or what to do with the findings. In addition, they often report that they have difficulty performing linguistic analyses, such as identifying different types of words (e.g., particles versus prepositions; participles versus gerunds; finite versus nonfinite verbs), sentences (e.g., simple versus complex; complex versus compound), and clauses (e.g., main, relative, adverbial, nominal) and in calculating various units of measurement (e.g., clausal density, mean length of utterance, mean length of C-unit, mean length of T-unit).

This book addresses these and other issues and provides sets of exercises to enhance learning or review. It also offers suggestions for designing intervention goals and activities to promote adolescents' use of complex language. After reading this book and completing the exercises, speech-language pathologists should be able to elicit, transcribe, and analyze language samples with adolescents quite successfully. They should also know what to do with that information to plan meaningful, relevant, and engaging intervention activities for adolescents.

A NOTE TO INSTRUCTORS

When this book is used as a text for university courses in language assessment and intervention, it is suggested that students be assigned to read chapters from Part II: Grammar Review and Exercises, while they are reading chapters from Part I: Working With Adolescents. This would provide students the opportunity to review grammar in manageable chunks before they are expected to apply the information to analyze a language sample. Note that the chapters in Part II build upon each other. For example, by covering word types (e.g., noun, verbs, adjectives) in Chapter 10 before clause types (e.g., nominal, adverbial, relative) in Chapter 11, students will understand how different types of words are similar to different types of clauses (e.g., nouns and nominal clauses; adjectives and relative clauses). Moreover, by covering clause types (e.g., main, coordinate, subordinate) before sentence types (e.g., simple, compound, complex) in Chapter 12, they will understand how the type of sentence is determined by the type(s) of clause(s) it contains. Finally, by covering sentence types before units of measurement (Chapter 13), students will be able to distinguish between complete and incomplete C-units and T-units and to determine whether a "run on" sentence is actually one, two, or three C-units or T-units.

Thus, it is suggested that during the first half of a semester, students be assigned to read the chapters in this sequence: 1 and 10, 2 and 11, 3 and 12, and 4 and 13 and 14. It is also recommended that class time be spent discussing their answers to the grammar review exercises. Then, during the second half of the semester, they could read the following chapters: 5, 6, 7, 8, and 9. Following this sequence, students would be prepared to elicit, transcribe, and analyze language samples from adolescents with typical or impaired language development during the second half of the course. The experience of conducting a language sample then will help to prepare them to apply their findings as they read and discuss the three chapters on language intervention (Chapters 7, 8, and 9).

—Marilyn A. Nippold

Acknowledgments

This book was completed with the support of many family members, friends, colleagues, and students. It was supported financially by the University of Oregon through the Hedco Foundation, a Hope Baney Faculty Award, and a Summer Faculty Award. Funding for some research projects was provided by the National Institute on Deafness and Other Communication Disorders (NIH), Grant 2P50DC02746-06A1; and the US-Israel Binational Science Foundation. Sincere gratitude is expressed to all.

This book is dedicated to Gary for all your support, love, and commitment.

PART I

Working With Adolescents

CHAPTER 1

Why Language Sampling?

*T*he ability to use language to express oneself with clarity, precision, and confidence in social, academic, and vocational settings is a basic human right. In our modern information-driven world in which effective and effortless communication is the standard expectation for all citizens, individuals who experience difficulties with spoken or written language—during formal or informal situations—are seriously hampered in their pursuit of personal satisfaction, independent living, and economic prosperity.

At least 10% of adolescents have language disorders that restrict their ability to express themselves verbally. This includes, for example, students with specific language impairment (SLI), nonspecific language impairment (NLI), learning disabilities, autism spectrum disorders (ASD), and traumatic brain injury (TBI; e.g., Bishop & Donlan, 2005; Landa & Goldberg, 2005; Lewis, Murdoch, & Woodyatt, 2007; Marinellie, 2004; Moran & Gillon, 2010; Moran, Kirk, & Powell, 2012; Nippold & Hesketh, 2009; Nippold, Mansfield, Billow, & Tomblin, 2008, 2009; Scott & Windsor, 2000; Ward-Lonergan, 2010; Ward-Lonergan, Liles, & Anderson, 1999). Frequently, students with these conditions exhibit limitations in their use of complex syntax, literate vocabulary, appropriate pragmatics, language content, and in their overall language productivity. Regarding syntax, adolescents with language disorders often produce shorter and simpler utterances than their peers with typical language development (TLD). Although some adolescents with language disorders also make errors on verb tenses, plurals, and pronouns (Scott, 2004), for the most part, they have mastered grammatical morphology but continue to struggle to produce complex sentences with adequate subordination (Nippold et al., 2008, 2009). Regarding the lexicon, many adolescents have difficulty understanding and using literate vocabulary such as abstract nouns, morphologically complex words, metacognitive verbs, and figurative expressions. During social situations, pragmatic issues may arise where they have difficulty answering questions, staying on topic, and showing sensitivity to other peoples' perspectives. Moreover, the content of their discourse may be impoverished, and they may be less productive speakers and writers than their peers with TLD.

In recent years, much has been learned about typical language development during adolescence and about the nature of language deficits experienced by some adolescents (Berman, 2004, 2008; Berman & Nir, 2010; Nippold, 2007; Paul & Norbury, 2012). Armed with a clear understanding of typical language development, speech-language pathologists can examine adolescents' abilities to communicate in natural settings by eliciting and analyzing spoken and written language samples and using the results to establish appropriate intervention goals. Standardized language tests such as the *Clinical Evaluation of Language Fundamentals-Third Edition* (Semel, Wiig, & Secord, 1995) are helpful in identifying language deficits (Nippold et al., 2009). However, they sample language out of context and do not provide the type of naturalistic information that is required to plan relevant intervention activities. Language sampling can help the speech-language pathologist address these limitations, focusing on the language of the curriculum and specific aspects of later language development, including complex syntax, the literate lexicon, and pragmatics. Language sampling also offers greater ecological validity than standardized language testing. Some of the many benefits of language sampling are listed in Table 1–1.

This book addresses language sampling in four essential genres: conversational, narrative, expository, and persuasive discourse. A conversation is a dialogue in which people take turns expressing their ideas, making comments, and asking questions in a spontaneous fashion. Because the goal of a conversation often is to establish, build, or maintain a relationship, speakers tend to support each other by acting as scaffolds, helping to expand or clarify what is being said. During the years between 10 and 18, young people spend increasing amounts of time in conversations with peers—in person or on the telephone—sharing information, building solidarity, and helping each other to solve complex problems (Nippold, 2007). The ability to use language to convey subtle and sophisticated thoughts to peers is essential for an adolescent's social development, self-esteem, personal identity, and overall well-being (Schickedanz, Schickedanz, Forsyth, & Forsyth, 2001).

The interactive nature of conversations makes them more supportive than other genres such as narrative, expository, or persuasive discourse in which the speaker is engaged in more of a monologue and bears most of the responsibility for communicating in a clear and efficient manner. Nevertheless, these other genres also are critical for social development, as when an adolescent tells stories to entertain a peer (narrative), explains to a classmate how to complete an assignment (expository), or tries to convince a friend to assist with a community project (persuasive).

TABLE 1–1. Some Benefits of Language Sampling with Adolescents

- The results of a language sample can indicate how well the adolescent communicates in "real-world" settings:
  - Conversing with others on the phone or in person
  - Telling stories to entertain a group of friends
  - Giving an oral report in history class
  - Explaining to a peer how to play a game or sport
  - Convincing a senior citizen to vote for a school bond
- During cognitively challenging speaking tasks, a language sample can reveal weaknesses in the use of complex syntax and the literate lexicon:
  - Frequent use of simple or incomplete sentences with little subordination
    - "You deal the cards. Take your turn. Pay a fine."
    - "You throw it to first base. Get the guy out."
    - "It's about two guys. One's bad."
  - Frequent use of imprecise, vague, or concrete words
    - "You play the song with this guitar-type thing."
    - "I don't know what it's called, but it's small and round."
    - "Our team needs stuff. We don't got enough."
- Difficulties with pragmatics can be observed, especially during conversations
  - Frequent interruptions and overlaps
  - Off-topic comments
  - Lack of empathy, sensitivity, awareness
  - Failure to consider others' perspectives
- Language productivity may be low in spoken or written language
  - Adolescent produces fewer words and utterances
  - Content is inaccurate, limited, or otherwise impoverished
- The results can supplement the findings of a standardized test.
  - Adolescent uses short, simple utterances
  - Adolescent produces grammatical errors
  - Adolescent uses vague, imprecise vocabulary
- The results can offer direction for intervention, focusing on:
  - Language needed to succeed socially, in school, and on the job
  - Appropriate pragmatic behaviors
  - Use of complex syntax and literate vocabulary
    - Subordinate clauses (relative, adverbial, nominal)
    - Subordinate clauses embedded within other subordinate clauses
    - Abstract nouns (e.g., ambition, strategy, expectation)
    - Morphologically complex words (e.g., availability, philanthropic)
    - Metacognitive verbs (e.g., determine, surmise, perceive)
    - Figurative expressions (metaphors, similes, idioms, proverbs)

Beyond the social uses of language, adolescents in today's schools are expected to use spoken and written language to meet state-mandated educational standards or benchmarks and to excel in the classroom.

Speech-language pathologists who work in middle schools and high schools frequently are called upon to address adolescents' spoken and written language skills. Working collaboratively with classroom teachers, many speech-language pathologists tailor their assessment and intervention activities to assist adolescents to meet specific Common Core State Standards (CCSS) for English Language Arts (National Governors Association Center for Best Practices and Council of Chief State School Officers, 2010; http://www.corestandards.org). According to the CCSS, beginning in grade 6 and continuing through grade 12, students are expected to demonstrate increasing levels of spoken and written language proficiency. Regarding spoken language, examples of school standards include the ability to "participate effectively in a range of conversations and collaborations with diverse partners, building on others' ideas and expressing their own clearly and persuasively" (p. 48). In addition, they are expected to "present information, findings, and supporting evidence such that listeners can follow the line of reasoning" (p. 48). Similarly, regarding written language, school standards include the ability to produce persuasive and expository essays that are clear, coherent, organized, logical, and supported by evidence, and to produce narrative essays that convey real or imaginary events with proper sequencing, structure, and detail. Given the key role that spoken and written language plays in school success, it is critical that speech-language pathologists have the appropriate knowledge and tools to assess and intervene effectively regarding conversational, narrative, expository, and persuasive discourse.

In addition to CCSS in speaking and writing, teachers place their own high expectations on students on a daily basis in the classroom. For example, regarding narrative discourse, the language of storytelling, a 5th-grade teacher may ask the class to read, retell, and discuss (orally or in writing) a folk tale such as *The Baker's Neighbor*, which concerns a conflict between an angry shopkeeper and a cheerful customer (Afflerbach, Beers, Blachowicz, Boyd, & Diffily, 2000). The story contains many abstract words (e.g., disbelief, fragrance, pleasures, privilege), and the characters express contrasting values and personality traits (e.g., greed, selfishness, contentment, honesty). To perform these activities, students must understand the story and its characters, including their actions, perspectives, and motivations. This requires that students listen, read, speak, and write proficiently. As students progress through grade levels, classroom expectations become even higher. In high school, for example, English teachers may require students to read, retell, and discuss the fable by Jean de La Fontaine, *The Value of Knowledge* (McDougal Littell, 2006). This story, a comment on pretentious and excessive wealth, concerns two citizens who represent contrasting values—one who is wealthy but rude and arrogant (the boor) and another who is poor but witty and humble (the bookman/wit). The fable concludes with the following literate lines:

> Our bookman doesn't deign respond: There's much too much that he might say. But still, revenge is his, and far beyond mere satire's meager means. For war breaks out and Mars wreaks havoc round about. Homeless, our vagabonds must beg their bread. Scorned everywhere, the boor meets glare and glower; welcomed, the wit is plied with board and bed. So ends their quarrel. Fools take heed: Knowledge is power! (p. 543)

Adolescents with language disorders are likely to be challenged mightily by this literate activity as they attempt to retell the fable and make sense of its low-frequency words (e.g., deign, revenge, satire, meager, plied), figurative expressions (e.g., beg their bread, knowledge is power), and uncommon syntactic structures (e.g., revenge is his, and far beyond mere satire's meager means; Mars wreaks havoc; plied with board and bed). For example, if asked to interpret the characters' actions, a student might reasonably be expected to use complex syntax and literate vocabulary, as in the following sentence:

> Although one of the characters in the story, the boor, is wealthy, people do not enjoy spending time with him because he is rude and arrogant.

Expository discourse, the use of language to convey information, is the most common genre used in the upper grades. Although narrative discourse predominates during the early grades, when students reach the 4th grade, a transition occurs in which expository discourse becomes the standard genre of the classroom (Nippold & Scott, 2010). At that time, teachers begin lecturing about complex topics in areas such as science, social studies, geography, mathematics, and history, and students' textbooks are written primarily in a direct, informative manner. In turn, students must display their knowledge of this newly acquired information through oral reports, group presentations, formal essays, and other assignments in which expository discourse is the expected genre. For example, consider the following excerpt from a 5th-grade science textbook:

> Scientists have classified plants into two main groups. Vascular plants, such as ferns and trees, have tubes. Because they have tubes to carry water, nutrients, and food, vascular plants can grow quite tall. Nonvascular plants, such as mosses, do not have tubes. So water must move from cell to cell. These plants need to live in a moist place, and they do not grow to be very large. (Jones et al., 2002, p. A53)

After reading about different classifications of plants and listening to their teachers' lectures, students are asked to write an expository essay in which they do the following:

Gather several types of plants, and examine their characteristics. Write clues describing each plant. Your clues can be about color, smell, height, size, or the plant's use, or they may tell where it was found. Read your clues to your classmates, and see if they can guess your plant. (Jones et al., 2002, p. A53)

As students progress through middle school and high school, the complexity of their reading and writing assignments becomes even greater, as illustrated by the following excerpt from a textbook used to teach American government in high school:

John Marshall (Chief Justice of the United States) set precedents that established important powers of the federal courts. Marshall served as Chief Justice of the United States from 1801 until 1835. As a Federalist, he established the independence of the judicial branch. In *Marbury v. Madison*, Marshall claimed for the Supreme Court the power to declare a law unconstitutional, and he affirmed the superiority of federal authority under the Constitution in *McCulloch v. Maryland* and *Gibbons v. Ogden*. In *McCulloch v. Maryland*, he wrote:

> This provision is made in a constitution, intended to endure for ages to come, and consequently, to be adapted to the various crises of human affairs. (McClenaghan, 2005, p. 81)

After learning about this American statesman, students are asked to do the following:

Write a paragraph explaining the meaning of Marshall's words in this quotation. Use information from your reading of the text to support your answer. (McClenaghan, 2005, p. 81)

Although both of these expository examples call upon the ability to use and understand complex syntax and difficult vocabulary, the high school example is more challenging because the sentences are longer, contain greater amounts of subordination, and use a greater number of low-frequency words expressing abstract concepts (e.g., precedents, independence, branch, superiority, authority, provision, ages, crises, affairs).

Persuasive discourse, language used to convince others to perform some action or to adopt a certain belief, is another prominent genre in today's middle school and high school classrooms. To illustrate, 5th-grade students learning about nutrition in science class may be asked to debate the issue of eating only plants versus eating both plants and animals. In debating this issue, they may be asked to offer reasons for and against both types of diets—vegetarian and omnivorous—before drawing their own conclusions (Jones et al., 2002, p. A113). To perform this activity successfully, students may need to gather information not only from their textbooks, but also from library books, science journals, newspapers, the Internet, and knowledgeable adults such as organic farmers.

High school students are expected to debate even more complex issues, such as the U.S. Supreme Court case of *Shelley v. Kraemer* that questioned the rights of individuals versus states to discriminate against people based on race or color. As a learning activity, students might be asked to "review the constitutional grounds on which each side based its arguments; to debate the opposing viewpoints; and to predict the impact of the Court's decision on discrimination" (McClenaghan, 2005, p. 677).

Beyond the classroom, proficiency with these genres is often called upon in the workplace where, in today's world, many adolescents have part-time jobs after school, on weekends, or during the summer months that require the ability to speak proficiently. For example, an adolescent who works at a daycare center may be asked to tell entertaining stories to young children; one who works at a recreation center may be asked to explain how to play an unfamiliar game; one who volunteers for a political party may be expected to convince fellow citizens to vote for a bond measure supporting education; and one who works in a veterinarian's office may be asked to explain an important health care procedure to a pet owner over the telephone, speaking in the following manner.

> Dr. Jones will be able to examine Zoe at six o'clock this evening. In the meantime, please keep her calm and comfortable, remove all food and water, and wrap her leg in a clean, dry towel before bringing her into the clinic.

Examples of other jobs that would require an adolescent to use complex language include explaining to a customer why the brakes on her road bike need to be replaced (while working as a bicycle mechanic), or describing the highlights of an historic town to a group of senior citizens (while working as a tour guide). Adolescents who can rise to the occasion during these sorts of speaking tasks are more likely to perform their jobs successfully.

Given the importance of verbal communication, this book offers guidelines for eliciting, transcribing, and analyzing spoken and written language samples in adolescents. Although language sampling as a formal activity has enjoyed a long history in our field (see Chapter 2), its use with adolescents has been quite limited. Nevertheless, this situation should improve as more information becomes available. The book also discusses intervention goals and activities, based on the results of a language sample. For adolescents with language disorders, intervention designed to enhance communication skills in conversational, narrative, expository, and persuasive discourse can lead to greater success in social, academic, and vocational endeavors, particularly when the intervention activities are cognitively stimulating, motivating, and relevant to their daily lives. When intervention focuses on the use of complex syntax and literate vocabulary, adolescents will be able to communicate with greater clarity, precision, and efficiency. Moreover, when it also addresses critical pragmatic issues, adolescents will be able to speak with greater confidence and poise.

Although few speech-language pathologists would disagree with these goals, we often have to "make the case" with administrators and policy makers as to why adolescents should receive speech-language services. After all, they often argue, if adolescents are still struggling with language disorders, isn't it too late to intervene? The resolute answer is, "No, it's not too late to help these young people!" (Nippold, 2010b). They are in a critical period of human development, transitioning from childhood to adulthood, moving from concrete to abstract thought, and preparing for the complexities of life in the 21st century as self-sufficient and contributing members of society. What happens now can "make or break" them, and fortunately, the speech-language pathologist, collaborating with classroom teachers, can assist adolescents to begin to gain traction and move forward with their spoken and written language skills.

Throughout this book, adolescents' use of complex syntax is emphasized in assessment and intervention. The reason for this emphasis is that syntax is the structural foundation of language (Crystal, 1996). As such, it enables an individual to express an infinite number of ideas. In particular, complex thought requires the use of complex syntax for efficient communication, evidenced by the following sentence, which contains two relative [REL] clauses, one adverbial [ADV] clause, and one main clause [MC]:

> Athletes who train [REL] in weather that is [REL] unusually warm need [MC] extra fluids throughout the day so that they will avoid [ADV] hyperthermia.

An emphasis on syntax also reflects the perspective that language proficiency is a basic human right. Given that we live in an information-driven world in which clear and effective communication is the standard expectation for all citizens, any difficulties with language can hamper the pursuit of independent living, economic prosperity, and personal satisfaction. Additionally, poor communication skills are a major source of strife and turmoil, and a substantial barrier to harmonious relationships. What better reasons can there be to support our efforts to promote language development in adolescents?

To convince any remaining skeptics of the importance of providing effective language intervention to adolescents—and of the benefits of eliciting language samples—the final section of this chapter presents excerpts from samples that were elicited from adolescents with typical and impaired language development (Tomblin & Nippold, 2014). Each adolescent was asked to perform the same task, to explain some key strategies needed to succeed at the sport of football. Each excerpt is coded for all main and subordinate clauses, and the results are discussed in order to illustrate how language sampling with adolescents can reveal individual strengths and weaknesses.

The first speaker is a 14-year-old boy with TLD (Tomblin & Nippold, 2014, p. 103):

> Make [MC] sure your teammates know [NOM] the play.
>
> And don't argue [MC] with your teammates.
>
> Because if you're arguing [ADV] with a lineman, the lineman could let [MC] the guy get [INF] by and you could get [MC] drilled.
>
> So your linemen are [MC] a big part of the game.
>
> You want [MC] your linemen in all of your plays.
>
> You want [MC] your linemen to feel [INF] good about themselves and their job because it doesn't seem [ADV] like they do [NOM] a lot.
>
> They just block [MC] the guy.
>
> But if nobody was [ADV] there, the running backs would get [MC] nowhere.
>
> And it helps [MC] to have [INF] a good lineman, and a good running back that can block [REL], and a halfback that can block [REL], and receivers that can catch [REL] and know [REL] their routes well, and just a team that doesn't fight [REL] and argue [REL] about everything. (44 words)
>
> If you mess [ADV] up, then just do [MC] better next time or try [MC] harder.

This excerpt contains 10 utterances and 149 words, and has a mean length of utterance (MLU) of 14.90 words. With 12 main clauses and 15 subordinate clauses, its clausal density (CD) is 2.70 clauses. Informal analysis suggests that the speaker has a strong knowledge base, reflected in his appropriate use of football terminology (e.g., lineman, halfback, running back, receiver) and relevant figurative expressions (e.g., get drilled, mess up). Syntactically, many of his sentences are complex, and the longest one, at 44 words, contains seven subordinate clauses. In addition to these lexical and syntactic strengths, pragmatic strengths include an awareness of the thoughts, feelings, and roles of the different players and of the negative consequences when team members cannot work together harmoniously.

The next speaker is a 14-year-old boy with SLI (Tomblin & Nippold, 2014, p. 103):

> You have [MC] to wear [INF] pads because when you're hit [ADV], it hurts [ADV].
>
> They have [MC] to work [INF] together and get [INF] the ball down the field.
>
> You pass [MC] the ball.

And you run [MC] the ball so you can get [ADV] to the end zone to score [INF].

You have [MC] to know [INF] how to kick [INF].

Because if you get [ADV] to the fourth down, you have [MC] to punt [INF] the ball away if you're [ADV] not ready to make [INF] it.

With 6 utterances and 73 words, this excerpt has an MLU of 12.17 words. It also contains 6 main clauses and 13 subordinate clauses, giving it a CD of 3.17 clauses. These numbers indicate that the production of complex sentences is a relative strength for this adolescent. He also uses a number of football terms and expressions (e.g., end zone, fourth down, run the ball) appropriately and shows an awareness of the need for team members to work together. However, in contrast with his peer with TLD (Speaker #1), his sample is sparser in terms of the amount of information it conveys, perhaps reflecting a more limited knowledge of football. There is also less variety in the types of nouns, verbs, and subordinate clauses that he employs.

The third speaker is a 13-year-old boy with NLI (Tomblin & Nippold, 2014, p. 103):

You should be [MC] a team player.

Like motivate [MC] your team to win [INF], not to fight [INF].

Have [MC] good sportsmanship.

Don't criticize [MC] or put [MC] down other teammates.

Be [MC] kind to other teammates.

Work [MC] as a team.

Encourage [MC] other people.

Be [MC] kind to your coaches.

This speaker's excerpt is much sparser than the other two, and with its 8 utterances and 43 words, it has an MLU of only 5.38 words. Although it contains 9 main clauses, there are only 2 subordinate clauses, reflecting a preponderance of simple sentences and a CD of only 1.38 clauses. The speaker therefore shows significant limitations in the use of complex syntax. Nevertheless, some strengths include the use of metalinguistic verbs (motivate, criticize, encourage) and an abstract noun (sportsmanship), and an awareness of the importance of working with teammates and coaches in a cooperative and friendly manner.

In sum, these three excerpts demonstrate how the speech-language pathologist can gain insight into the unique strengths and weaknesses that individual speakers display in their production of language, information that can be used to plan meaningful and relevant intervention activities for adolescents. This is especially true when the speech-language pathologist has a strong background in the nature of later language development, is familiar with the spoken and written language demands of contemporary classrooms, and is able to work intensely with students and collaboratively with teachers and other school professionals in those classrooms.

CHAPTER 2

History of
Language Sampling

*L*anguage sampling has a long tradition in the field of speech-language pathology. Table 2–1 highlights certain events in the history of language sampling. Modern language sampling can be traced back to the late 19th century with the publication of the first diary studies. These were longitudinal studies conducted by parents—often linguists, psychologists, or other scientists—who carefully observed and described their own children's language development, beginning in infancy and continuing into childhood. The data typically consisted of handwritten notes and direct quotations of the child, playing alone or interacting with family members in everyday situations. Hippolyte Taine (1877) published one of the earliest studies, describing his daughter's early development. Charles Darwin (1877), Milton Humphreys (1880), and William Preyer (1889) soon followed with similar reports of their own children's development.

Diary studies continued into the 20th century. For example, Werner Leopold, a professor of English at Northwestern University, wrote a four-volume series (Leopold, 1939–1949) on the language development of his daughter Hildegard, who was acquiring both English and German. Although most diary studies have focused on the first few years of life, the account of Hildegard's development covered the years from birth through adolescence, and it is one of the most detailed and well-known studies ever reported. However, in the absence of audio recorders, diary studies were limited in the amount of language that could be recorded, particularly after the child had moved beyond the single-word stage and was speaking rapidly and in multiword utterances. Thus, the reports of Hildegard's language, for example, consisted mainly of summaries of her behavior

TABLE 2–1. History of Language Sampling

- 19th century
  - Diary studies begin, with focus on early development of typical children
    - Taine (1877)
    - Darwin (1877)
    - Humphreys (1880)
    - Preyer (1889)
- 20th century
  - Diary studies continue, e.g., Leopold (1939–1949)
  - Formal language sampling begins
    - Smith (1926)
    - McCarthy (1930)
    - Templin (1957)
  - Invention of the tape recorder (Wikipedia, 2009)
    - "Blattnerphone" (L. Blattner, Germany, 1929; Wikipedia, 2009)
    - "K1" (F. Matthias, Germany, 1935; Wikipedia, 2009)
    - Both had poor sound quality
    - Ampex Electronics Company of California developed high-quality tape recorder for singer Bing Crosby (1947; Wikipedia, 2009).
  - Chomsky's influential books are published: *Syntactic Structures* (1957) and *Aspects of the Theory of Syntax* (1965)
  - Researchers use tape recorders to collect language samples longitudinally
  - Emphasis is placed on the development of syntax in young children
  - Interest in determining underlying linguistic rules or "competence"
    - Braine (1963)
    - Miller & Ervin (1964)
    - Bloom (1970)
    - Brown (1973)
    - de Villiers & de Villiers (1973)
  - Formal language sampling programs are published
    - Developmental Sentence Scoring (DSS; Lee, 1974)
    - Language Sampling, Analysis, & Training (LSAT; Tyack & Gottsleben, 1974)
    - Language Assessment, Remediation, and Screening Procedures (LARSP; Crystal, Fletcher, & Garman, 1976)
    - Assessing Language Production in Children (Miller, 1981)
    - Language Sample Analysis: The Wisconsin Guide (Leadholm & Miller, 1992)
    - Guide to Analysis of Language Transcripts (Retherford, 1993)
    - Strong Narrative Assessment Procedure (SNAP; Strong, Mayer, & Mayer, 1998)
  - Developmental studies include older children and adolescents (e.g., Hunt, 1970; Loban, 1976)

TABLE 2–1. *continued*

- o Developmental studies examine written language as well as spoken language (Hunt, 1970; Loban, 1976)
- o Interest in persuasive discourse emerges and expands
  - ▪ Spoken persuasion
    - • Wood, Weinstein, & Parker (1967)
    - • Flavell, Botkin, Fry, Wright, & Jarvis (1968)
    - • Bragg, Ostrowski, & Finley (1973)
    - • Finley & Humphreys (1974)
    - • Clark & Delia (1976)
    - • Piche, Rubin, & Michlin (1978)
    - • Bearison & Gass (1979)
    - • Delia, Kline, & Burleson (1979)
    - • Ritter (1979)
    - • Jones (1985)
    - • Erftmier & Dyson (1986)
  - ▪ Written persuasion
    - • Crowhurst & Piche (1979)
    - • Rubin & Piche (1979)
    - • Crowhurst (1980, 1987, 1990)
    - • Kroll (1984)
    - • McCann (1989)
    - • Knudson (1992)
    - • Wong, Butler, Ficzere, & Kuperis (1996)
- o Interest in narrative discourse emerges and expands
  - ▪ Botvin & Sutton-Smith (1977)
  - ▪ Kernan (1977)
  - ▪ Stein & Glenn (1979)
  - ▪ Roth & Spekman (1986)
  - ▪ Liles (1985, 1987, 1993)
  - ▪ Merritt & Liles (1987, 1989)
  - ▪ Scott (1988)
  - ▪ Bamberg & Damrad-Frye (1991)
  - ▪ Liles, Duffy, Merritt, & Purcell (1995)
- o Computer programs are designed to analyze language samples
  - ▪ Systematic Analysis of Language Transcripts (SALT; Miller & Chapman, 1983)
  - ▪ Child Language Analysis Program (CLAN; MacWhinney, 1988)
  - ▪ Computerized Profiling (Long & Fey, 1993)

continues

TABLE 2–1. *continued*

- 21st century
  - Widespread use of digital recorders and microcassettes
  - Interest in narrative discourse continues to expand
    - Scott & Windsor (2000)
    - Windsor, Scott, & Street (2000)
    - Berman & Verhoeven (2002)
    - Verhoeven et al. (2002)
    - Justice et al. (2006)
    - McCabe, Bliss, Barra, & Bennett (2008)
    - Ukrainetz & Gillam (2009)
  - Interest in adolescent language expands (Nippold, 2007)
  - Normative databases expand (e.g., Miller, 2009)
  - New language sampling programs are published for school-age children, emphasizing narrative discourse
    - Expression, Reception, and Recall of Narrative Instrument (ERRNI; Bishop, 2004)
    - Test of Narrative Language (TNL; Gillam & Pearson, 2004)
  - Persuasive discourse is examined in children, adolescents, and adults
    - Felton & Kuhn (2001)
    - Nippold, Ward-Lonergan, & Fanning (2005)
    - Nippold & Ward-Lonergan (2010)
  - New focus on examining expository discourse in adolescents
    - Scott & Windsor (2000)
    - Berman & Verhoeven (2002)
    - Verhoeven et al. (2002)
    - Nippold, Hesketh, Duthie, & Mansfield (2005)
    - Nippold, Mansfield, & Billow (2007)
    - Nippold, Mansfield, Billow, & Tomblin (2008)
    - Nippold, Mansfield, Billow, & Tomblin (2009)
    - Nippold (2009)
    - Nippold & Scott (2010)

(e.g., at age 10: "Hildegard finds difficulty in telling me about her experiences in coherent German narration," Vol. 4, p. 148) and isolated quotations (e.g., at age 14: "Oh Papa, don't speak German in the street," Vol. 4, p. 153). Despite their limitations, diary studies offered insights into the complex and creative nature of language development, sparking broad interest in it as a serious topic of scientific investigation. Further information on diary studies is available in Ingram (1989) and Behrens (2008).

During the 1920s, researchers began to conduct cross-sectional studies of language development by examining large numbers of children at different ages (Ingram, 1989). For example, Smith (1926) studied 124 children (ages 2–5 years); McCarthy (1930) studied 140 children (ages 1–4 years); and Templin (1957) studied 430 children (ages 3–8 years). In those studies, samples of conversational speech were elicited from each child and often analyzed for the mean number of words per utterance. However, rather than using audio recorders to collect the samples, researchers wrote down the children's utterances as they were speaking (Ingram, 1989). Given the large number of utterances that even young children can produce, the validity of their findings was questionable. Nevertheless, those early studies paved the way for later research that examined language development in greater detail, and Chomsky's (1957, 1965) work on transformational grammar prompted even more sophisticated studies (e.g., Bloom, 1970; Braine, 1963; Brown, 1973; de Villiers & de Villiers, 1973; Miller & Ervin, 1964).

INVENTION OF THE AUDIO RECORDER

It is intriguing to consider how the invention of the audio recorder helped to revolutionize the study of language development. In 1929, Ludwig Blattner, a German scientist, developed the "Blattnerphone" for recording human speech. Then, in 1935, Frederick Matthias developed the "K1," also in Germany. The sound quality of those early recorders was quite poor, and it was not until 1947 that Ampex Electronics Company of California developed a high-quality audio recorder for the American singer Bing Crosby. A perfectionist, Crosby wished to prerecord the songs that would be played on his radio shows. A shrewd businessman, Crosby invested in the company for large-scale commercial production of audio recorders (Wikipedia, 2009).

Eventually, audio recorders became available to the general public, including researchers and clinicians. This made it possible to establish valid databases of spoken language development in young children (e.g., Miller, 1981) and to study older children and adolescents (e.g., Loban, 1976), who present even greater challenges because of the amount and complexity of their spoken language. Figure 2–1 shows an excerpt from a language sample elicited from a toddler. Without being able to audio record this child's speech, one could probably write down most of her single-word utterances. However, even an expert transcriber would have difficulty keeping up with her when she begins to produce successive multiword utterances. Now consider the adolescent in Figure 2–2. Given the sophisticated nature of her oral language, it would be virtually impossible to transcribe her speech without a reliable audio recorder! Of course, many researchers and clinicians now use microcassettes, including digital versions, for recording language samples.

Girl—Age 17 Months

- juice juice
- allgone
- gimme wawa
- pwease!
- whatdat?
- doggie!
- kitty go!

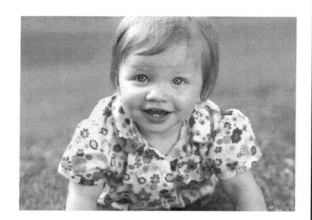

FIGURE 2–1. Early utterances, relatively easy to transcribe by hand. (Camille Tokerud/Photographer's Choice RF/Getty Images)

Girl—Age 17 Years

Q: Why is track and field your favorite sport?

A: Well I had a knee injury my freshman year playing volleyball. And I couldn't do a lot of running. And in track and field, I can be a thrower, which is in the field events, and not have to do a lot of running, and work at my own pace, and not have to compete with other students, just competing to better yourself. So you don't have to say, "Oh well, they're better than me so I can't be as good as them."

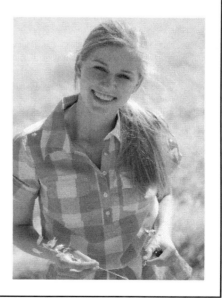

FIGURE 2–2. Adolescent talk, impossible to analyze without an audio recorder. (PT Images/Getty Images)

FORMAL LANGUAGE SAMPLING PROGRAMS

By the 1970s, language sampling had become a widely recommended clinical tool for examining children's language development (e.g., Bloom & Lahey, 1978; Lynch, 1978; Trantham & Pedersen, 1976; Wiig & Semel, 1976; also see Launer & Lahey, 1981, for further discussion). Consistent with this recommendation, a number of formal programs were published, offering guidelines for speech-language pathologists on how to elicit, transcribe, and analyze samples of conversational speech. Several well-known programs are listed in Table 2–1. They include, for example, *Developmental Sentence Scoring* (DSS; Lee, 1974), *Language Sampling, Analysis, & Training* (LSAT; Tyack & Gottsleben, 1974), and *Language Assessment, Remediation, and Screening Procedures* (LARSP; Crystal, Fletcher, & Garman, 1976). Additional programs were developed in the 1980s and 1990s, including those by Miller (1981), Leadholm and Miller (1992), and Retherford (1993). Those programs were designed to identify a young child's linguistic weaknesses, thereby providing direction for intervention. For example, if a language sample showed that a 4-year-old child omitted certain grammatical classes (e.g., articles, conjunctions), or used grammatical morphemes inconsistently (e.g., past tense -*ed*, plural -*s*), intervention would be designed to increase the frequency with which the child used those forms correctly in spontaneous speech (Launer & Lahey, 1981). This method of using language samples to identify grammatical weaknesses and other communication deficits and to develop relevant goals for intervention continues to be recommended (Paul & Norbury, 2012).

Since the 1980s, researchers and clinicians who have studied language development or have designed or used clinical tools for language sampling have been assisted greatly by the invention of software packages that have increased the speed, accuracy, and efficiency of this enterprise. Well-known examples include *Systematic Analysis of Language Transcripts* (SALT; Miller, 2009; Miller & Chapman, 1983, 2003), *Child Language Analysis Program* (CLAN; MacWhinney, 1988), and *Computerized Profiling* (Long & Fey, 1993). Without those computer-assisted programs, we might still be analyzing language samples by hand. SALT has been especially helpful to the field because it has been continuously updated since its beginning and now includes a bilingual Spanish/English version (http://www.languageanalysislab.com/).

BEYOND CONVERSATION

In the field of speech-language pathology, there is a strong tradition of eliciting language samples in conversational speech for individuals of all ages (e.g., Larson & McKinley, 2003; Lee, 1974; Loban, 1976; Nelson, 1998;

Paul, 2007; Templin, 1957; Tyack & Gottsleben, 1974). However, during the 1970s, interest in studying children's ability to tell stories—to employ narrative discourse—began. Given the complex nature of narratives, those early studies often included older children and young adolescents (e.g., Botvin & Sutton-Smith, 1977; Kernan, 1977; Stein & Glenn, 1979).

Interest in studying narrative discourse continued during the 1980s and 1990s (e.g., Berman & Slobin, 1994; Eder, 1988; Hadley, 1998; Klecan-Aker & Caraway, 1997; Leadholm & Miller, 1992; Liles, 1985, 1987, 1993; Liles, Duffy, Merritt, & Purcell, 1995; Merritt & Liles, 1987, 1989; Roth & Spekman, 1986; Scott, 1988) and has remained strong during the 21st century (e.g., Berman & Verhoeven, 2002; Justice et al., 2006; McCabe, Bliss, Barra, & Bennett, 2008; Nippold, Frantz-Kaspar, Cramond, Kirk, Hayward-Mayhew, & MacKinnon, 2014; Scott & Windsor, 2000; Sun & Nippold, 2012; Ukrainetz & Gillam, 2009; Windsor, Scott, & Street, 2000). Researchers thus have been prompted to design language sampling programs specifically for narrative discourse such as the *Strong Narrative Assessment Procedure* (SNAP; Strong, Mayer, & Mayer, 1998). More recent tools have been published by Bishop (2004) and Gillam and Pearson (2004). However, because none of the available tools were designed specifically to examine narrative ability in adolescents, Nippold et al. (2014) designed a new task for adolescents involving fables (see Chapter 5). It was important to design a narrative task for adolescents because storytelling is often called upon in social, academic, and vocational contexts. Moreover, samples of narrative speaking tend to elicit greater syntactic complexity than samples of conversational speech in children and adolescents (Leadholm & Miller, 1992; Nippold et al., 2014), and are therefore more likely to reveal a speaker's linguistic competence than are conversational samples.

In recent years, interest in examining other genres besides conversational and narrative discourse has grown. In particular, the importance of persuasive and expository discourse has been recognized (e.g., Nippold & Scott, 2010; Nippold & Ward-Lonergan, 2010; Nippold, Ward-Lonergan, & Fanning, 2005), because research has shown that genre makes a difference in the complexity of language that a speaker or writer produces. Just as samples of narrative discourse can elicit greater syntactic complexity than samples of conversational discourse (Leadholm & Miller, 1992; Nippold et al., 2014), samples of expository and persuasive discourse can elicit greater syntactic complexity than samples of conversational and narrative discourse in speakers of all ages (Berman & Verhoeven, 2002; Crowhurst, 1980; Crowhurst & Piche, 1979; Nippold, Cramond, & Hayward-Mayhew, 2013; Nippold, Hesketh, Duthie, & Mansfield, 2005; Scott & Windsor, 2000; Verhoeven et al., 2002).

The importance of expository discourse is underscored by the finding that samples elicited in this genre are more likely to reveal both strengths and weaknesses in adolescents' syntax compared with samples of conversational discourse (e.g., Nippold & Sun, 2010; Nippold, Hesketh, Duthie, &

Mansfield, 2005; Nippold, Mansfield, & Billow, 2007; Nippold, Mansfield, Billow, & Tomblin, 2008, 2009). To illustrate this point, Table 2–2 contains excerpts from the conversational samples of two adolescents. Speaker #1 is a 15-year-old boy with typical language development, and Speaker #2 is a 14-year-old boy with autism spectrum disorder. For Speaker #1, the mean length of C-unit (MLCU) for his entire conversation was only 5.38 words. Although he responded politely to the interviewer's questions, his sentences were short, with little elaboration. Speaker #2 produced an MLCU of 7.17, slightly higher than that of Speaker #1. However, many of his utterances were fragments and did not meet criteria for a C-unit, which consists of a main clause and any subordinate clauses attached to it. Then, during an expository task in which the speakers talked about the game of chess, each boy's level of syntactic complexity increased dramatically, illustrated by the excerpts contained in Table 2–3. For example, when Speaker #1

TABLE 2–2. Excerpts from the Conversational Samples of Two Adolescents (from the Author's Files)

Speaker #1, a 15-year-old boy with typical language development (MLCU = 5.83 words)

Q: Do you have any brothers or sisters?

A: Yes, I have two brothers.

Q: What are their names?

A: My older brother is named Andrew. And my younger brother is named Ross.

Q: How old are they?

A: Andrew is 19. Ross is 9.

Q: What else can you tell me about them?

A: Well, Ross is hyperactive. And Andrew lives on his own now. And he doesn't return calls very often.

Speaker #2, a 14-year-old boy with autism spectrum disorder (MLCU = 7.17 words)

Q: Do you have a favorite TV show or movie?

A: Not really. I don't really watch TV much. I mostly play video games rather than watch TV or movies.

Q: What kind of video games do you play?

A: Um, usually Black Saturday games. It's like strategy type games.

Q: Do you like to read books or magazines?

A: Books, not magazines. Books just like the adventure types. Like not mysteries but just like adventure.

TABLE 2–3. Excerpts from the Expository Samples of the Same Adolescents Shown in Table 2–2 (from the Author's Files)

Speaker #1, a 15-year-old boy with typical language development (MLCU = 19.83)

And then there is the knight, which moves in an "L" shape, which is really good at forking pieces, like attacking two different pieces at the same time so that they have to lose one of them. Because its movement is so irregular, nothing but another knight can really stop it. Then there is the rook, which can move horizontally or vertically. And they tend to be really useful because you can put a rook behind a pawn and march the pawn down the board to try to get a queen. And the rook will be defending it the entire time.

Speaker #2, a 14-year-old boy with autism spectrum disorder (MLCU = 10.39)

It's good to learn some defensive strategies to try to arrange your pieces in ways that they are hard to crack, like hard to get through and break through. Then you have to always stay on the offensive because other people will play off of you. And just keep advancing over and over and over. And offensive, you have to be kind of defensive. And the same time, you study your moves and try thinking several moves ahead.

---

explained to an adult how various chess pieces move, the MLCU for his entire sample was 19.83. Similarly, when Speaker #2 explained to an adult some key strategies needed to win a game of chess, the MLCU for his entire sample was 10.39. Had the speech-language pathologist not elicited the expository samples in addition to the conversational samples, the syntactic competence of these two adolescents might not have been revealed.

Like expository discourse, persuasive discourse offers the potential to reveal linguistic competence as when students are asked to take a position about a controversy (e.g., "Should animals be trained to perform in circuses?") and to write a convincing essay in which they describe and defend their views. During such tasks, developmental gains in syntax, semantics, and pragmatics can be documented (Nippold, Ward-Lonergan, & Fanning, 2005). Examples include the use of relative clauses, abstract nouns, metacognitive and metalinguistic verbs, and the ability to view a controversy from multiple perspectives.

Nevertheless, as discussed throughout this book, it is important to elicit samples of conversational, narrative, expository, and persuasive discourse in adolescents, because all four genres can provide useful information to a speech-language pathologist. For example, conversational samples can reveal limitations in pragmatics, the social use of language. Narrative, expository, and persuasive samples can reveal limitations in the use of complex syntax, weaknesses that may not be apparent in general conversation (Nippold, Mansfield, Billow, & Tomblin, 2008).

Hence, it is expected that in the years ahead, researchers and clinicians will continue to investigate discourse development and to design innovative techniques for eliciting, transcribing, and analyzing language samples in all four genres. The goal will be to utilize that information to design new methods of enhancing adolescents' ability to communicate with clarity, precision, and confidence in spoken and written language.

CHAPTER 3

Adolescent Language Development

Adolescence is a stage in human development when young people are transitioning from childhood to adulthood, moving from concrete to abstract thought, and preparing for the challenges of living as independent, self-sufficient, responsible, and contributing members of society. Consistent with this growth in cognition and autonomy, research in neuroscience has shown that the brain continues to mature during adolescence and into adulthood, particularly in the frontal-temporal regions that are responsible for executive functioning (Savage, 2009).

Language development during adolescence is characterized by gradual and protracted growth in all major domains, including syntax, semantics, and pragmatics. Syntactically, sentences become longer and contain greater amounts of subordination, a change that is often measured in terms of mean length of C-unit (spoken language) or T-unit (written language). A C-unit or T-unit consists of one main clause and any attached subordinate clauses (Hunt, 1970). However, C-units, unlike T-units, also may include answers to questions that are incomplete sentences (Loban, 1976). Mean length of utterance (MLU) also is used to measure syntactic development during adolescence (e.g., Miller, 2009), in which utterances include full sentences as well as shorter productions in spoken or written language.

During adolescence, gains also occur in the use and understanding of literate words such as abstract nouns, adverbial conjuncts, metacognitive verbs, and morphologically complex nouns and adjectives. Pragmatically, adolescents show gains in interpersonal skills such as listening attentively while others are speaking, and entertaining their peers with amusing anecdotes (Nippold, 2007; Schickedanz, Schickedanz, Forsyth, & Forsyth, 2001). Tables 3–1, 3–2, and 3–3 list some of the major changes that occur in language development during adolescence.

TABLE 3–1. Syntactic Development During Adolescence (Nippold, 2007)

- Sentences gradually increase in length and complexity
- Increased sentence length is achieved through:
  - Greater use of subordinate clauses
    - Relative (Athletes *who train in the heat* may suffer hyperthermia.)
    - Nominal (The club required *that everyone plant a tree.*)
    - Adverbial (*If you don't wash your hands*, you might get sick.)
  - Multiple levels of subordination occur within sentences (hierarchical complexity, e.g., athletes who train in weather that is unusually warm need extra fluids throughout the day so that they will avoid hyperthermia).
- Use of subordination allows for greater efficiency and precision in speech
- However, utterance length and complexity vary with genre:
  - Narrative > Conversational
  - Expository > Narrative
  - Expository > Conversational
  - Persuasive > Narrative
  - Persuasive > Conversational
- Other factors affect length and complexity of utterances:
  - Topic knowledge
  - Topic interest
  - Motivation to talk
- Greater use of low-frequency syntactic structures, for example:
  - Appositives (What he wanted, *a sports car*, was in the driveway.)
  - Elaborated noun phrases (*Instruments such as banjos, dulcimers, and fiddles* are played in Appalachia.)
  - Subject postmodification via prepositional phrase (The mountains *to the east* are the Cascades.)
  - Clefting (*It was 1951* when the 22nd Amendment was adopted.)
  - The passive voice (Hypothermia *is caused by exposure to extreme cold.*)
  - Greater use of cohesive devices within and across sentences
    - Subordinate conjunctions (although, before, since, unless, whenever)
    - Coordinate conjunctions (also, and, but, or, so)
    - Adverbial conjuncts (e.g., however, therefore, moreover, consequently)

TABLE 3–2. Semantic Development During Adolescence (Nippold, 2007; Santrock, 1996)

- Greater use and understanding of figurative language
  - Idioms (Hang on one's coattails, keep the pot boiling.)
  - Metaphors and similes (Anticipation is a magnifying glass of coming events; his mind was locked like the jaws of an angry shark.)
  - Proverbs (Gentleness skillfully subdues wrath.)
  - Slang expressions (da bomb, fave, no brainer, preps)
- Greater use and understanding of humor, wit, satire, and sarcasm
  - Tells funny jokes and amusing anecdotes
  - Engages the listener with dramatic storytelling
- Greater use and understanding of literate vocabulary
  - Abstract nouns (anticipation, chaos, mystique, spectrum, triumph)
  - Adverbial conjuncts (moreover, similarly, conversely, rather)
  - Metacognitive verbs
    - Factive (ascertain, comprehend, determine, recognize)
    - Nonfactive (assume, doubt, judge, suppose)
  - Metalinguistic verbs (confess, declare, inquire, pronounce)
  - Technical terms (carbon dioxide, oxygen, photosynthesis)
  - Morphologically complex words:
    - Derived nominals (concealment, dictatorship, tactfulness)
    - Derived adjectives (algebraic, consolable, merciful)

Although the focus of this book is on adolescence, it should be noted that language development in each of these areas continues well into adulthood.

Underlying this growth in language are significant changes in cognitive, social, and emotional development, as adolescents move into formal operational thought, a stage that is characterized by the ability to reason hypothetically, to speculate about possibilities beyond the present, and to solve problems in a logical and systematic fashion (Santrock, 1996). During adolescence and early adulthood, there is also a growing awareness of other peoples' thoughts, feelings, and beliefs, which influences social communication (Schickedanz et al., 2001). Growth in the knowledge base, obtained through education and world experience, also influences language development in adolescents and young adults (Santrock, 1996). Table 3–4 lists some highlights of cognitive and social-emotional development that occur during adolescence.

TABLE 3–3. Pragmatic Development During Adolescence (Nippold, 2007; Schickedanz, Schickedanz, Forsyth, & Forsyth, 2001)

- Conversations with peers increase in frequency and offer a new source of information, emotional support, and personal well-being.

- Talking in person and talking on the telephone increase.

- Electronic communication increases (e.g., e-mail, text-messaging).

- Improvements occur in conversational discourse.
  - Asks relevant questions
  - Interrupts appropriately
  - Makes factually related comments
  - Makes supportive comments
  - Shifts topics gracefully
  - Takes perspectives of others
  - Takes turns and allows others to talk
  - Uses body language and facial expressions
  - Uses discretion and good judgment with personal information
  - Uses humor and figurative expressions to entertain

- Improvements occur in narrative discourse.
  - Produces original and detailed stories
  - Takes perspectives of others
  - Entertains listener with dramatic storytelling

- Improvements occur in expository discourse.
  - Employs perspective-taking to explain
  - Adjusts to needs of listener
  - Shows greater knowledge of topic

- Improvements occur in persuasive discourse.
  - Generates variety of arguments to convince another
  - Anticipates counterarguments of listener
  - Focuses on needs and interests of the listener to convince
  - Considers merits of opposing points of view

Some of the changes in language development can be illustrated by comparing two essays written by girls with typical language development, who were writing about friendship (from the author's file). The first example was produced by a 10-year-old girl:

TABLE 3–4. Cognitive and Social-Emotional Development During Adolescence (Santrock, 1996; Schickedanz et al., 2001)

- Cognitive development
  - Thinks abstractly, creatively, flexibly, imaginatively
  - Understands issues from multiple points of view
  - Holds multiple variables in mind simultaneously
  - Shows interest in complex social, political, and philosophical issues
  - Uses logic to solve science problems
  - Approaches problems in systematic, organized fashion
  - Generates hypotheses, reasons deductively
  - Organizes and integrates varied pieces of information

- Social-emotional development
  - Understands other people's thoughts, feelings, and beliefs
  - Uses metacognition to analyze own behavior, feelings, beliefs
  - Shows increased interest in spending time with peers
  - Seeks close friendships and feelings of solidarity
  - Seeks independence from family yet maintains closeness
  - Searches for personal identity (e.g., career, politics, religion)
  - Experiences dating and romantic relationships
  - Achieves stability in personality traits (e.g., extroversion versus introversion; agreeableness versus disagreeableness)

> People can become friends by playing a game or being a science partner and more. Boys can ruin a friendship. Also you could get in a terrible fight and wind up with bruises, broken bones, or bloody noses.

Note that she has used only one abstract noun (friendship) and no metacognitive verbs. The next example, produced by a 17-year-old girl, is more advanced in that it contains 5 abstract nouns (level, trust, values, time, friendship) and two metacognitive verbs (trust, hold), reflecting a more sophisticated way of thinking about the topic. In addition, her sentences are longer and more complex, with each containing an adverbial clause:

> People can become good friends *when a level of trust is developed. When you can trust a person to hold the values you do, are accepting, and do the best thing for you*, your time is more often spent with them. *When this trust is damaged*, the friendship can be in danger.

Information concerning normal development provides a solid foundation for examining the communication skills of adolescents who have been identified as having language disorders. For example, when analyzing language samples produced by adolescents, it is important to determine MLCU (or MLTU) and clausal density, which is the total number of main and subordinate clauses divided by the total number of C-units (or T-units) produced. Although both of these measures gradually increase during adolescence and into adulthood, adolescents with language disorders often show marked deficits in these areas (Nippold, Mansfield, Billow, & Tomblin, 2008, 2009). One also should note the presence of literate vocabulary (Scott, 2010) such as abstract nouns and metacognitive verbs, for these types of words also may be problematic for adolescents with language disorders.

It is important to examine these later developing phenomena because they can allow a speaker to communicate more efficiently. For example, rather than producing a monotonous string of simple sentences (e.g., "Friendship is important. You trust someone. They accept you. So you spend time with them."), the proficient language user can integrate multiple thoughts into one complex sentence that is easier to process (e.g., "Friendship is important because it brings trust, acceptance, and companionship."). It is important also to identify specific types of subordinate clauses, because they each enable a speaker to perform unique functions. For example, adverbial clauses allow one to express conditions, reasons, and temporal relationships (*if you need me on Saturday*, I'm available to babysit; she went to the party *because she wanted to meet new people*; *before you go home*, please take some candy). Relative clauses allow one to describe nouns that are in subject or object position (e.g., the car *that gets the best gas mileage* will be the most popular; the students studied in the library *that stayed open all night*). Nominal clauses allow one to describe mental or verbal events (e.g., the teacher decided that *she would grade the exams*; the students argued that *they should receive higher grades*).

The overlap between syntax and the lexicon also should be noted. In proficient language users, each type of subordinate clause is associated with a different set of words. For example, adverbial clauses co-occur with subordinate conjunctions (before, until, unless); relative clauses co-occur with abstract nouns (the *claim* that you made; the *trust* that she sought); and nominal clauses co-occur with metacognitive (believe, know, wish) and metalinguistic (say, tell, whisper) verbs. As discussed in Chapters 7, 8, and 9, this type of information can be useful in designing language intervention for adolescents.

CHAPTER 4

Language Sampling Guidelines

When evaluating the language skills of an adolescent, a well-designed norm-referenced test such as the *Clinical Evaluation of Language Fundamentals-Fifth Edition* (Semel, Wiig, & Secord, 2013) should be used to identify the presence of a language disorder. After a disorder has been documented, language sampling should be used to determine how well the adolescent speaks in a variety of natural communication settings. Importantly, language sampling should be used as a supplement to norm-referenced testing, not as a substitute for it. This is because well-designed norm-referenced tests have greater reliability and validity than language-sampling tasks. Factors that affect the reliability and validity of language samples are discussed in this chapter.

Listed in Table 4–1 are a number of challenges associated with language sampling in adolescents. One concern is that a speaker's performance is influenced greatly by psychosocial factors. These include the speaker's knowledge of the topic, motivation to talk about it, and the degree to which the interviewer's questions stimulate complex thought. When speakers are well informed about the topic, interested in discussing it, and presented with stimulating prompts, their performance is likely to be quite strong. Genre is another factor that influences performance with studies showing that greater syntactic complexity occurs during expository discourse compared with narrative or conversational discourse (Berman & Verhoeven, 2002; Nippold, 2009; Nippold, Hesketh, Duthie, & Mansfield, 2005; Scott & Windsor, 2000). Another concern is the paucity of normative data for language sampling tasks with adolescents. Until this latter problem is addressed through large-scale research, language sampling should be used informally to obtain naturalistic information about how an adolescent

TABLE 4–1. Some Challenges Associated with Language Sampling in Adolescents

---

- Performance is influenced by psychosocial factors
  - Is the adolescent knowledgeable of the topic?
  - Is the adolescent motivated to talk?
  - Do the interviewer's questions stimulate complex thought?
  - Performance varies with genre, with greater syntactic complexity in:
    - expository than in narrative discourse
    - expository than in conversational discourse
    - persuasive than in narrative discourse
    - narrative than in conversational discourse
- Normative data for adolescents is quite limited
  - New tasks (narrative, expository, and persuasive) must be designed
  - Large-scale studies to develop normative databases are needed
    - Mean length of C-unit/T-unit
    - Types of subordinate clauses
    - Clausal density
    - Productivity (total utterances, total words)
    - Use of literate words (abstract nouns, metacognitive verbs, morphologically complex words, adverbial conjuncts)

---

communicates and to establish relevant goals for intervention, as discussed later in this book. Some key factors to analyze are listed in Table 4–2. Language productivity and syntactic complexity are emphasized because these areas are often problematic for adolescents with language disorders.

The ultimate goal of language intervention with adolescents is to improve their ability to communicate in meaningful contexts beyond the borders of the therapy room. This includes, for example, the diverse social, academic, and vocational settings that they encounter today as adolescents and will encounter tomorrow as adults. Given these expectations, it is reasonable to focus on intervention activities that will generalize to those settings, emphasizing the need for adolescents to use spoken and written language in a way that is clear, precise, and efficient. By eliciting, transcribing, and analyzing language samples, speech-language pathologists can gain insight into the unique strengths and weaknesses that an adolescent exhibits in different situations. Although language sampling is not a perfect process, the information obtained can be used to establish relevant goals for intervention and to monitor change as the adolescent achieves greater accuracy, precision, efficiency, and confidence when communicating with others for genuine purposes.

TABLE 4–2. Key Factors to Analyze in Adolescent Language Samples

---

- Total utterances produced, a measure of language productivity
- Total words produced, a measure of language productivity
- Mean length of C-unit/T-unit, a measure of syntactic complexity
- Clausal density, a measure of syntactic complexity
- Specific types of subordinate clauses produced
  - Nominal [NOM]
    - She explained *that he prefers waffles over pancakes.*
    - I believe *Topalov will win the tournament.*
  - Relative [REL]
    - He just beat Topalov, *who was the best in the world.*
    - The rider *who won the Tour de France that year* was from Italy.
  - Adverbial [ADV]
    - I learned chess *when I was three years old.*
    - The rook can move horizontally or vertically *as much as it wants.*
- Instances of subordinate clauses embedded within other subordinate clauses (hierarchical complexity):
  - If a piece takes [ADV] out the piece that has [REL] the king in check, I can take out that piece. (Here, the REL is embedded within the ADV.)
  - So if I had [ADV] like a castle and a bishop up here, which is [REL] the one that can move [REL] on a diagonal, I can kind of like protect it. (Here, the second REL is embedded within the first REL, which in turn, is embedded within the ADV.)

Before presenting specific tasks that can be used to elicit language samples with adolescents (see Chapter 5), I offer some general guidelines for eliciting, transcribing, and analyzing language samples, especially when spoken language is being examined.

GENERAL SUGGESTIONS

During the language sampling interview, the speech-language pathologist should encourage the adolescent's best performance in order to reveal both strengths and weaknesses. This can be accomplished by attending to *confidentiality* and *interaction style* (Table 4–3).

Regarding confidentiality, the speech-language pathologist should explain that the purpose of the activity is to learn about the adolescent in order to obtain information that will be useful in planning intervention.

TABLE 4–3. Guidelines for Eliciting Spoken Language Samples with Adolescents

---

Confidentiality

- Conduct the interview in a quiet, private area, free of distractions.
- Explain the purpose of the activity.
- Explain how the information will be used.
- Obtain the adolescent's permission (in writing).
  - To be interviewed
  - To be audio-recorded
- Ensure discretion in what the adolescent says.
- Encourage questions from the adolescent.
- Answer questions honestly.

Interaction Style

- Convey respect and genuine interest in the adolescent.
- Listen patiently through lengthy or confusing discourse.
- Remain calm, attentive, and upbeat.
- Avoid arguments with the adolescent.
- Avoid interruptions and overlaps of speech.
- Use appropriate eye contact and body language.
- Make supportive and positive comments.
- Ask open-ended questions.
- Ask one question at a time.
- Pause after asking a question (count to four silently).
- Repeat or rephrase a question, as necessary.
- Feel free to "go with the flow" to encourage spontaneity.
- Use humor, as appropriate (good natured, kind, nonoffensive).

The speech-language pathologist should obtain the adolescent's written permission to conduct the session and to audio-record the interview, asking him or her to sign a consent form. The adolescent should be assured that whatever is discussed during the interview will not be shared with others. Questions should be encouraged and answered honestly.

During the interview, the importance of the speech-language pathologist's *interaction style* cannot be overemphasized. To reveal the adolescent's strengths, the speech-language pathologist must show genuine respect for the adolescent and his or her feelings, attitudes, and beliefs. This can be accomplished by taking time to listen patiently; to remain calm, attentive, and upbeat; to avoid arguments, interruptions, and overlaps of speech; and to show interest through appropriate eye contact, body language (e.g., smiling, nodding), and supportive comments (e.g., "Uh-huh," "I know what you mean," "Tell me more"). It is critical also to pause (e.g., count to four silently) after asking a question to allow the adolescent time to formulate a reply. Although verbal interaction in today's world is often fast-paced and competitive, with speakers and listeners quick to fill the silence, speech-language pathologists need to use a more relaxed style of interaction with adolescents, one that is kind, puts the young person at ease, and shows that the speaker's comments matter. Interjecting a bit of humor into the session also may help the adolescent feel more comfortable speaking with the speech-language pathologist.

Regarding the interaction, it is important for the speech-language pathologist to follow a structured protocol that includes questions that were designed to elicit certain types of information in a particular genre (e.g., conversational or expository). However, in addition to following the protocol, the speech-language pathologist should feel free to "go with the flow" and to ask follow-up questions that will encourage the adolescent to continue speaking, to elaborate on an idea, and to communicate freely and confidently. In other words, the interviewer should attempt to promote a more natural interaction style with the adolescent.

Speech-language pathologists frequently ask how many utterances they should attempt to elicit when interviewing an adolescent. Research has not yet determined an ideal number of utterances. The best rule of thumb may be, "the more the better" in order to obtain a representative sample. Realistically, however, this is not always practical, and meaningful results can be obtained with fewer than the standard 50 to 100 utterances that are often recommended (e.g., Miller, 1981). Rather than attempting to reach a certain minimum, it is more important to encourage the adolescent to talk by bringing up stimulating topics, asking open-ended questions, showing genuine interest, and following the other suggestions for interacting with adolescents, as described previously.

In addition to issues of confidentiality and interaction style, some important points regarding the use of technology and the transcription of the interview must be addressed so that the language sampling activity is maximally productive. These points are listed in Table 4–4. Although many of them may seem obvious, too often they are forgotten, leading to frustration and wasted time and effort.

For example, regarding technology, the speech-language pathologist should practice using the recording equipment in advance and making sure that everything is working properly before starting the interview.

TABLE 4–4. Key Points Regarding the Spoken Language Sampling Session

Using Technology

- Ensure that the environment is quiet and free of distractions.
- Use a good quality audio recorder (digital or analog).
- If using an analog tape recorder, employ a high-quality audiotape.
- Adjust the volume of the audio recorder before starting the interview.
- Turn on the recorder and ask the adolescent speaker to count to 10.
- Immediately replay the recorder to ensure proper volume and clarity.
- If necessary, adjust the distance between the speaker's mouth and the microphone.
- Restart the audio recorder before beginning the formal interview.

Transcribing the Sample

- Transcribe the sample as soon as possible after eliciting it. When the sample is fresh in mind, it is easier to transcribe accurately.
- Transcribe the sample verbatim, with all mazes and errors included.
- Enter each new utterance on its own line.
- Go back later and parenthesize all that constitutes maze behavior.
- If using SALT, all mazes will automatically be disregarded.
- Run-on sentences should be broken up so that main clauses linked by coordinate conjunctions, such as *and, but,* and *or,* each begin a new utterance. The following utterance, even though spoken continuously, would be broken at the slashes:

    My parents went to Portland for the weekend / but I stayed with my cousin in Creswell / and my brother went camping with a friend.

- Two or more main clauses spoken continuously without a pause and without a conjunction (e.g., "I don't know how to braid hair my friend did this," "It's a potluck bring your favorite dish") are broken into multiple utterances as follows:

    I don't know how to braid hair.
    My friend did this.
    It's a potluck.
    Bring your favorite dish.

Using SALT

- Place each new utterance on its own line.
- Put parentheses around all mazes, allowing the final reformulation to stand.
- To code clause types, place the code type in brackets, one space after its verb, using codes such as MC (main clause), ADV (adverbial clause), REL (relative clause), or NOM (nominal clause).
- To code word types, place the code in brackets with no space after the word, using codes such as [ABN] (abstract noun) or [MCV] (metacognitive verb).
- This will enable SALT to create separate lists for clauses and words

To illustrate this point, a speech-language pathologist recently set up an interview with an adolescent at his high school, after having gone through a lengthy process of gaining permission from the school district, the boys' parents, and the boy himself in order to obtain a language sample for a research project. She arrived at the school well before the appointment, checked in with the head secretary, and set up the audio recorder in a quiet room near the main office. The interview with the adolescent went extremely well, with the speech-language pathologist eliciting a lively, detailed, and intriguing sample of expository discourse. However, upon returning home and attempting to transcribe the sample, she discovered that she had pushed the wrong button on the audio cassette and that nothing had been recorded, to her great dismay! Unfortunately, it was impossible to return to the school and redo the interview. I share this story, hoping it will help others attend to important details, knowing that it is the little things in life that often make a big difference.

Language samples with adolescents can be analyzed effectively after they have been transcribed and entered into the software program, *Systematic Analysis of Language Transcripts* (SALT; http://www.languageanalysis lab.com/). SALT can be adapted to allow the user to code various types of clauses (e.g., main and subordinate). In addition, SALT will automatically calculate Mean Length of C-unit (MLCU), Mean Length of T-unit (MLTU), or Mean Length of Utterance (MLU), as discussed. Regarding the *transcription*, it is important to listen to the recording carefully and to type the adolescent's utterances exactly as they were produced, with all mazes (i.e., false starts, repetitions, and revisions) included. Parentheses should be placed around mazes, allowing the final reformulation to stand. Any words included within parentheses will not be counted when SALT calculates the mean number of words per utterance (C-unit/ T-unit) for the sample. With practice, the speech-language pathologist will be able to transcribe directly into SALT, placing each new utterance on its own line. Some professionals prefer initially to transcribe the sample into Microsoft Word and then to transfer it to SALT. However, this is an extra step that can be avoided with further practice.

After entering a sample, the speech-language pathologist can go back over it and identify instances of main and subordinate clauses, using codes such as [MC] (main clause), [ADV] (adverbial clause), and [NOM] (nominal clause). All codes should be enclosed in brackets. When clauses are coded, the code should follow the verb and be separated by one space. Table 4–5 contains portions of a language sample that was entered into SALT and coded in this manner. When coding words, such as abstract nouns or metacognitive verbs, the code (e.g., [ABN], [MCV]) should immediately follow the word, with no space. By using these conventions, SALT will automatically tabulate the number of times that each type of clause or word occurred in the sample and will create separate lists of clause types (e.g., MC, REL, ADV, NOM) and word types (e.g., ABN, MCV). It is important to

TABLE 4–5. Excerpt from an Expository Language Sample That Has Been Entered into SALT and Coded for Main and Subordinate Clauses

---

All mazes are enclosed in parentheses. The speaker (C), a 17-year-old girl, is explaining how to play baseball.

    MC = main clause

    ADV = adverbial clause

    REL = relative clause

    INF = infinitive clause

    PRT = participial clause

C (or if you just) As soon as you hit [ADV] the ball, you have [MC] to run [INF] to first.

C And if the ball gets [ADV] to first before you do [ADV], then you're [MC] out.

C And (there's the pitch for) when you're pitching [ADV], there's [MC] four balls and three strikes.

C If you get three strikes on you [ADV], (you) you're [MC] out.

C If you get [ADV] four balls, you get [MC] to walk [INF] to first base.

C And (for each for third base) for first base, there's [MC] dropped third strike.

C Like if the pitcher pitches [ADV] it and you screen [ADV] but the first base doesn't catch [ADV] it, the person batting [PRT] can run [MC] to first.

C But if you fouled [ADV] it like (if it) if the batter hits [ADV] it and it goes [ADV] (like) out of where you're playing [REL], then that's [MC] a foul ball.

---

know that SALT can be adapted to perform any type of coding function, depending on the interests of the speech-language pathologist. The codes discussed in this book are those that were used in several recent research projects. Part II of this book contains exercises for identifying various types of words, phrases, clauses, sentences, and units of measurement that are important for analyzing adolescent language. To obtain a copy of SALT and to learn more about using it, the reader is referred to their website at the University of Wisconsin, Madison (http://www.languageanalysislab.com).

CHAPTER 5

Language Sampling Tasks

*T*his chapter presents a set of language-sampling tasks that were used in a series of recent investigations (Nippold, 2009; Nippold, Frantz-Kaspar, Cramond, Kirk, Hayward-Mayhew, & MacKinnon, 2014; Nippold & Hesketh, 2009; Nippold, Hesketh, Duthie, & Mansfield, 2005; Nippold, Mansfield, & Billow, 2007; Nippold, Mansfield, Billow, & Tomblin, 2008, 2009; Nippold & Sun, 2010; Nippold, Ward-Lonergan, & Fanning, 2005; Sun & Nippold, 2012). The studies examined children, adolescents, and adults, focusing on the use of complex syntax in conversational, narrative, expository, or persuasive discourse. All tasks effectively elicited spoken or written discourse from individuals with typical or impaired language development.

CONVERSATIONAL DISCOURSE

During conversations, adolescents with typical and impaired language development produce utterances that are shorter and less complex than those they produce during other genres such as explanations (Nippold, 2009; Nippold, Hesketh, Duthie, & Mansfield, 2005; Nippold, Billow, Mansfield, & Tomblin, 2008). Although samples of conversational discourse are less likely to reveal deficits in syntactic development compared with samples of expository discourse (Nippold et al., 2008), it is important to elicit conversations because those sessions can help to build rapport with adolescents and can reveal relevant information about their attitudes, interests, and concerns. Moreover, during a conversation, the speech-language pathologist will have the opportunity to observe any pragmatic issues that might be challenging to the adolescent (e.g., difficulty answering questions, staying on topic, making eye contact). Finally, some adolescents with language impairments, such as those with ASD, do show deficits in the use of complex syntax during conversations (Nippold & Hesketh, 2009), as discussed in Chapter 6.

To elicit a conversational sample, it is recommended that the speech-language pathologist follow a structured protocol, such as the one shown in Table 5–1, which is called the *General Conversation* task. After asking a question, the speech-language pathologist should pause and allow the adolescent time to formulate a reply. When it appears that the adolescent has finished talking, the speech-language pathologist should feel free to comment on the adolescent's response and to ask additional questions to encourage elaboration, promoting a more natural interaction. Table 5–2 contains an excerpt from a conversation that took place between a speech-language pathologist and a 13-year-old girl with typical language development. It illustrates how the speech-language pathologist encouraged conversation by showing interest in what the girl said, asking topic-relevant questions, and making supportive comments. The sample has been coded for main and subordinate clauses.

After eliciting a general conversation, the speech-language pathologist may wish to elicit a conversation about a specific topic of interest, focusing on a favorite hobby or other activity. When conversing about topics of high personal interest, speakers are more likely to use complex syntax as compared with when they talking about topics they find less engaging (Nippold, 2009). As an example, the conversational task shown in Table 5–3 was used with speakers who were chess players, and it elicited greater syntactic complexity than did the general conversation task. The speech-language pathologist could easily change the topic of conversation from chess to any other hobby, depending on the interests of the adolescent (e.g., soccer, golf, tennis, ballet, cheerleading, volleyball) and could make other modifications to customize the interview for a specific activity. However, it is important to remember that eliciting conversation about such topics is quite different from eliciting an expository sample focusing on those same topics.

TABLE 5–1. General Conversation Task (Nippold, 2009, p. 860)

Interviewer: First of all, I'd like to learn something about you. I'm going to ask you a few general questions. Then you can ask me some questions, too. OK?

A. Do you have any brothers or sisters? (if yes) What are their names? How old are they? What else can you tell me about them?

B. Do you have any pets at home? (if yes) Tell me about your pets.

C. Do you have a favorite TV show or movie? (if yes) Tell me about it.

D. Do you like to read books or magazines? (if yes) Which ones?

E. Now do you want to ask me anything? (Allow 1–2 quick questions.)

TABLE 5–2. General Conversation Between 13-Year-Old Girl with TLD (C) and Examiner (E; from the Author's Files)

The sample has been coded for clause types: MC = main clause; ADV = adverbial clause; NOM = nominal clause; REL = relative clause; INF = infinitive clause; PRT = participial clause; GER = gerund clause.

Girl, Age 13, Conversing About General Topics of Interest (TCU = 30; MLCU = 8.77; CD = 1.37

E What would you like to tell me about yourself?

E For example, school, family, friends, pets, or your birthday?

C Well, last year, I started [MC] dance with some of my friends.

C And I decided [MC] to do [INF] it again this year.

C And I started [MC] last week.

C So far, it's been [MC] really fun.

C And last year, we did [MC] a show at the community center.

C And I liked [MC] it a lot.

C So I'm [MC] pretty excited about that.

E What do you dance, what style?

C I dance [MC] ballet, well, kind of contemporary.

C I do [MC] point on one day, modern on another day, and ballet on another one.

E So you perform all those types of dance per performance?

C Yeah, and we did [MC] the *Tempest* in a kind of dance form.

E Oh really?

E What is the *Tempest*?

C It's [MC] a Shakespeare play about these people who get [REL] shipwrecked on an island.

C And one of the persons on the island who is [REL] already there used [MC] to be [INF] a king.

C And his brother kicked [MC] him out or took [MC] over.

C And then his brother is [MC] the one who gets [REL] shipwrecked on the island.

C And then the first brother does [MC] all this stuff to him to pay [INF] back.

C But in the end, they make [MC] up.

C So it was [MC] all good.

E Do you feel like it was well represented in dance?

C Yeah, I think [MC] so.

C It was [MC] a lot of fun.

C And I can understand [MC] it, which is [REL] a good thing.

C And school just started [MC], eighth grade.

C And it's [MC] kind of weird being [GER] on the top, not having [GER] the other older kids there.

continues

TABLE 5–2. *continued*

C It's [MC] just strange.

C But I'm kind of getting [MC] used to it.

E Do you like it?

C Yeah, I like [MC] it.

E But it's only one year and then it's back to being a freshman again, next year.

C Yeah, that part isn't [MC] so great.

C And I talked [MC] to some of the people that are [REL] freshmen this year that I knew [REL] last year.

C And they say [MC] it's [NOM] pretty scary.

E Oh no!

C Yeah.

E But you have a lot of friends in your grade?

C Yeah.

E So you'll all go together.

TABLE 5–3. Chess Conversation Task (Nippold, 2009, p. 860)

Introduction: Now I'd like to ask you about chess:

A. How long have you played chess?

B. How old were you when you first started to play?

C. Who taught you how to play chess?

D. Do you have a chess rating? (if yes) What is it?

E. Do you have a chess coach or teacher? (if yes) Tell me about him or her.

F. Do you belong to a chess club? (if yes) Which one?

G. How often do you play chess, say, in a typical week?

H. Who do you play with the most?

I. Can you name any famous chess players? (if yes) Tell me something about him or her/them.

J. Do you ever play chess on a computer? Tell me about that.

K. Now tell me why you enjoy chess.

Table 5–4 contains an example of conversation about chess with a preadolescent boy. It can be seen that many of the boy's responses to the examiner's questions were short and to the point until he began talking about topics of greater personal interest. For example, when the boy talked about playing bughouse, playing chess on a computer, or why he enjoyed chess, the complexity of his language increased, revealing a fairly sophisticated level of syntactic development.

TABLE 5–4. Conversation About Chess Between the Examiner and a Preadolescent Boy, Age 9;10 (from the Author's Files) E = Examiner; C = Child

Boy, Age 9;10 Conversing about Chess (TCU = 41; MLCU = 7.32; CD = 1.41)

E How long have you played chess?

C About two years.

E And how old were you when you first started to play?

C Seven.

E And who taught you how to play chess?

C My friend.

C His name was [MC] Michael.

C And I think [MC] he was [NOM] 16 years old.

C Anything more you needed [REL] to ask [INF] me?

E Anything more you can tell me about Michael?

C (He umm started playing) I knew [MC] him when I was [ADV] first born because he was playing [ADV] with my older brother, Frank.

C And that is [MC] all I know [REL].

C And he still lives [MC] with his parents.

E Do you have a chess rating?

C I am [MC] first in club so far.

C I have not been beat [MC] for a while, except by my uncle.

C He is [MC] 19.

C He beat [MC] me just barely.

C And that is [MC] all.

E Do you belong to a chess club?

C Yes.

E Do you have a chess coach or teacher?

C Yeah, I have [MC] a chess teacher.

C But I do not know [MC] his name though because he is [ADV] new.

C Our old teacher had [MC] to move [INF].

C Yeah, I learned [MC] a lot from him.

E Can you tell me any more about him?

C (umm) He is [MC] usually late.

C And (umm) he has taught [MC] me a game.

C It is [MC] bughouse.

C It is [MC] when you are [NOM] on a team.

C And if you take [ADV] somebody's piece, if your partner takes [ADV] somebody else's piece, you get it [MC].

C And if you take [ADV] somebody else's piece, you give [MC] them that piece to them.

continues

TABLE 5–4. *continued*

C And they get [MC] to set [INF] it up anywhere else.

C They can set [MC] anywhere on the board they want [REL] except it has [ADV] to be [INF] on their side and the pawns cannot be [ADV] on the back.

C Anything else?

E How often do you play chess?

C About every day.

E So, who do you play with the most?

C My brother Timothy.

E Can you name any famous chess players?

C I do not think [MC] so.

E Okay, do you ever play chess on a computer?

C Yes, I got [MC] Chess_master, the 10th edition.

C And it is [MC] pretty challenging.

C And I have [MC] Battle_chess_III.

C And it is [MC] 3-D when you have [ADV] actually these real (umm) war pieces that you move [REL].

C And you can actually make [MC] them fight [INF].

C It is [MC] pretty cool.

E How often do you play on the computer?

C About every day.

E So you play a computer every day and you also play a person.

E Now tell me why you enjoy chess.

C It is [MC] a pretty challenging sport.

C And you have [MC] to know [INF] a bunch of strategies to basically know [INF] how to play [INF].

C And it is [MC] really fun to challenge [INF] people because you have [ADV] to use [INF] a bunch of mathematics.

NARRATIVE DISCOURSE

Narrative discourse, or storytelling, is commonly elicited in school-age children through wordless picture books such as *Frog, Where Are You?* (Mayer, 1969) in which the child examines the book and is asked to generate a story about the pictures and tell the story to the examiner (Bamberg, 1994; Berman & Slobin, 1994; Epstein & Phillips, 2009; McCabe et al., 2008). However, the juvenile nature of the stories renders them inappropriate for adolescents. Unfortunately, little research has focused on narrative development in adolescents, and for this reason, few tasks are available in the literature. Nevertheless, it is important to examine spoken and written narrative discourse in adolescents because this genre plays a prominent role in middle school and high school literature classes in which students are frequently asked to read, retell, interpret, and write narratives in the form of plays, short stories, folk tales, and fables. In addition, narratives often are used in social situations throughout the life span to entertain or comfort others.

Spoken Language

Given the shortage of narrative speaking tasks for adolescents, Nippold et al. (2014) created a task that involved the retelling of two fables, *The Mice in Council* and *The Monkey and the Dolphin*. Each fable was accompanied by a colorful illustration. The protocol used to present the stories and to elicit the retelling of each is shown in Table 5–5. Fables were used to elicit narrative speaking in adolescents because these stories, although superficially simple, deal with complex themes (e.g., pride, collaboration, honesty, pretense) that might be of interest to adolescents, given their cognitive, social, and emotional development. It was predicted that the abstract nature of the stories would prompt complex thought and therefore the use of complex syntax as the adolescents retold the fables. It was also predicted that syntactic complexity during narrative speaking would be greater than when the same adolescents were engaged in conversational speaking.

To examine these predictions, Nippold et al. (2014) individually interviewed 40 adolescents (20 boys and 20 girls; mean age = 14 years) who had typical language development and were native speakers of American English. Each narrative sample was transcribed verbatim, coded for the use of main and subordinate clauses, and examined for mean length of C-unit (MLCU) and clausal density (CD). Results of the study confirmed both predictions.

Table 5–6 contains an example of an adolescent girl's retelling of both fables. It can be seen that she produces a number of long and complex utterances that contain multiple levels of clausal embedding, as in the following example from the *Mice in Council*:

> And then one of the elder mice, who's obviously thought [REL] the solution out more than everybody else, (he says) he says [MC] this is [NOM] a great proposal but who is going [NOM] to put [INF] the bell on the cat?

A similar level of syntactic complexity occurs when she states the moral of the *Monkey and the Dolphin*:

> The moral was [MC] that if you pretend [ADV] to be [INF] something other than yourself, you might just find [NOM] yourself in deeper water than you were [ADV] before.

TABLE 5–5. Narrative Speaking Tasks Using Fables (Nippold et al., 2014)

(Interviewer reads the following slowly and clearly . . .)

"This is a storytelling activity that involves fables. Fables are imaginary stories about animals that act like people. I am going to read you two different fables. Please listen to each one carefully. Be ready to tell each story back to me, in your own words. Try to remember as much as you can, so that you can tell the whole story back to me. After you finish, I will ask you some questions about the story. There are no penalties for incorrect answers. I just want to know what you think about the stories. Are you ready? . . . Here's the first one."

SHOW FABLE CARD TO PARTICIPANT . . .

The Mice in Council

The mice lived in constant terror of the cat, whose greatest pleasure was toying with them and eating them up. The mice called a meeting to try to solve their problems. Many plans were discussed but none seemed right. What to do about the great cat?

At last a small mouse leaped up. He drew himself up to his full height. "I propose," he said, "that a bell be hung around the cat's neck so that whenever he approaches, we will hear the bell tinkle and we shall be able to escape." All the mice applauded, and the young mouse took a few bows and then sat down.

After the motion was seconded and passed, a wise old mouse slowly rose to his feet. "My friends, fellow mice, our young friend has proposed a brilliant solution to end our constant fear and jeopardy from the cat. Only a mouse of great genius could have conceived such a simple solution, for indeed with the bell around his neck, we shall all most certainly hear Mr. Cat's no longer stealthy approach. But one question occurs to this old head. Who, may I ask, shall bell the cat?"

Moral: Some things are easier said than done (Lawrence, 1997, p. 19).

Interviewer asks participant to retell the story. . . . (Turn on audio recorder)

TURN OVER CARD TO SHOW NEXT FABLE

"Here's the next story, the last one. Listen carefully and be ready to tell it back to me."

The Monkey and the Dolphin

It was an old custom among sailors to take with them on their voyages monkeys and other pets to amuse them while they were at sea. So it happened that on a certain voyage a sailor took with him a monkey as a companion on board ship.

Off the coast of Sunium, the famous promontory of Attica, the ship was caught in a violent storm and was wrecked. All on board were thrown into the water and had to swim for land as best they could. And among them was the monkey.

A dolphin saw him struggling in the waves, and taking him for a man, went to his assistance. As they were nearing the shore just opposite Piraeus, the harbor of Athens, the dolphin spoke. "Are you an Athenian?" he asked.

"Yes, indeed," replied the monkey, as he spat out a mouthful of sea water. "I belong to one of the first families of the city."

"Then, of course, you know Piraeus," said the dolphin.

"Oh yes," said the monkey, who thought Piraeus must be the name of some distinguished citizen, "he is one of my very dearest friends."

Disgusted by so obvious a falsehood, the dolphin dived to the bottom of the sea and left the monkey to his fate.

Moral: Those who pretend to be what they are not, sooner or later, find themselves in deep water (Grosset & Dunlap, 1947, pp. 198–199).

Interviewer asks participant to retell the story. . . . (Turn on audio recorder)

TABLE 5–6. Adolescent Girl's Retelling of Two Fables (from the Author's Files)

Note: Each retelling has been coded for clause types. TCU = total communication units; MLCU = mean length of C-unit; CD = clausal density; MC = main clause; NOM = nominal clause; ADV = adverbial clause; REL = relative clause; INF = infinitive clause; PRT = participial clause; GER = gerund clause.

Girl, Age 14;2

Retelling the Mice in Council (TCU = 12; MLCU = 11.92; CD = 2.17)

E Can you retell that story?

C Yeah, so the story is [MC] about a council of mice.

C And they're trying [MC] to figure [INF] out what they can do [NOM] about their problem.

C And their problem is [MC] that there's [NOM] a cat who takes [REL] advantage of them and plays [REL] with them and eats [REL] them.

C And that's [MC] obviously not good for the mice.

C So they're trying [MC] to think [INF] of a solution.

C And this little teeny mouse (he says) well he stands [MC] up.

C And he says [MC] let [NOM]'s put [INF] a bell around the cat's neck.

C And everybody's [MC] like, wow that's [NOM] amazing.

C (And the) and then (um they) they vote [MC] on it.

C And then (the) it passes [MC].

C So they're [MC] in agreement.

C And then one of the elder mice, who's obviously thought [REL] the solution out more than everybody else, (he says) he says [MC] this is [NOM] a great proposal but who is going [NOM] to put [INF] the bell on the cat?

E Nice.

E Thank you.

Retelling the Monkey and the Dolphin (TCU = 20; MLCU = 10.75; CD = 1.85)

E Can you retell the story?

C Kay, so there were [MC] (uh) sailors.

C And they were [MC] out on their ship with their pets.

C And (there) there was [MC] a storm.

C And (they got) they were stranded [MC] (I guess) in the middle of the sea.

C And (uh) they were all trying [MC] to swim [INF] back to shore.

C And some of them were probably drowning [MC] and stuff.

C And it was [MC] horrible.

C (And) and a dolphin came [MC] up to one of the pets and (uh) asked [MC] if he was [NOM] a citizen of Athens (I guess).

continues

TABLE 5–6. *continued*

C And (the) the monkey decided [MC] to play [INF] up to the dolphin cause he (I guess he uh) thought [ADV] (that) that (would make) the dolphin would obviously take [NOM] him to land and he'd be [NOM] safe.

C He'd (um) benefit [MC] from playing [GER] up the dolphin.

C And (uh) so the dolphin was asking [MC] him stuff.

C And (he was being) he was kind of boasting [MC] about it.

C And he was [MC] like oh yeah I'm [NOM] rich and famous.

C And then the dolphin asked [MC] him a pretty simple question.

C And he took [MC] it the wrong way.

C And it was [MC] obviously a lie because that's [ADV] not what it was [REL] (that's and um and).

C And the dolphin decided [MC] that he was [NOM] n't worth it because he was lied [ADV] to.

C (Um) (he wasn't) he wasn't [MC] truthful about himself (so).

E Nice.

C Do you want [MC] the moral?

E You can tell the moral, too.

C The moral was [MC] that if you pretend [ADV] to be [INF] something other than yourself, you might just find [NOM] yourself in deeper water than you were [ADV] before.

E Nice.

E Yeah, I really like the way you said that.

In sum, the results of the study indicate that fables can be an effective way of eliciting complex syntax in the narrative speaking of young adolescents. Future studies are needed to examine narrative speaking in adolescents with language impairments, using fables.

Written Language

To learn about the development of narrative production in older students, Sun and Nippold (2012) conducted a study in which 5th-grade children (mean age = 11 years old), 8th-grade adolescents (mean age = 14 years old), and 11th-grade adolescents (mean age = 17 years old; n = 40 per group) wrote essays at school in their classrooms. All students spoke Standard American English as their primary language and had typical language development (TLD). Titled "What Happened One Day," the essay requested them to write a story—factual or imaginary—about something funny, sad, or scary that happened to them and a friend. The students were given an outline that prompted them to address a set of story grammar elements. They also were given booklets of lined paper in which to write their stories, and they were allowed 20 minutes to complete each one. The task, as presented to the students, is shown in Table 5–7.

The results of the study indicated that the 11th graders outperformed the 8th and 5th graders on Total T-Units (i.e., sentences), a measure of language productivity, and that both the 11th and 8th graders outperformed the 5th graders on mean length of T-unit (MLTU), a measure of syntactic complexity. In addition, the 8th graders outperformed the 5th graders on clausal density, another measure of syntactic complexity. It was also found that the oldest group used a greater frequency of abstract nouns

TABLE 5–7. Narrative Writing Task, "What Happened One Day" (Sun & Nippold, 2012)

At this time, I would like you to write a story. Please write a story about something funny, sad, or scary that happened to you and a friend. You get to decide what to write about. It can be anything that was funny, sad, or scary. If you can't think of something that really happened, you can make it up. It doesn't have to be a true story. You can use your imagination, if you want. It's up to you.

The following outline will help you organize your thoughts and write a good story. In your story, be sure to do the following:

1. Tell where the events took place (the setting).
2. Tell who the main people are (characters).
3. Tell everything that happened in the story (plot).
4. Tell about the problems that came up (problems).
5. Explain what the characters tried to do (attempts).
6. Explain how things turned out (outcome).
7. Tell how everyone felt during the events (thoughts).

Keep this list of points in front of you as you write your story. As you address each point, try to write a full paragraph of your own ideas. You will have 20 minutes to complete your work. I have given you a booklet of lined paper to use in writing your story. Please put your name, age, and grade level on the booklet.

As you do this work, please use your best writing style with complete sentences and correct grammar, spelling, and punctuation. If you aren't sure how to spell a word, make your best guess. Try to write neatly, using a pen or pencil. If you make a mistake, just cross it out or use an eraser. Keep going until I ask you to stop writing.

Do you have any questions?

The title of your story is "What Happened One Day."

(e.g., *accomplishment, apathy, imagination*) and metacognitive verbs (e.g., *assume, reflect, ignore*) than did the youngest group. Importantly, all groups appeared to enjoy the narrative activity, with many of them requesting to continue writing their stories, even after the time limit was called. This pattern suggested that the task was interesting and motivating to the children and adolescents in this investigation.

Table 5–8 contains examples of two narrative essays produced by participants in the study, an 11-year-old boy (Writer #1) and a 13-year-old boy (Writer #2). For each writer, MLTU and Clausal Density (CD) are reported. In addition to finite clauses (MC, REL, NOM, ADV), all nonfinite clauses are coded in these examples and included as part of the Clausal Density calculation. Nonfinite clauses include infinitives (INF), gerundives (GER), and participles (PRT). Although the two boys performed similarly in terms of MLTU, the older boy produced a higher level of Clausal Density than did the younger one, reflecting a greater amount of subordination in his essay. In addition to examining the amount of subordination, it is important to consider the extent to which a writer produces multiple levels of subordination, or hierarchical complexity. This can be seen by comparing each writer's longest sentence. Those are as follows:

> *Writer #1:* Then we had [MC] to walk [INF] way down and around the whole outside of the whole huge mall. (17 words)

> *Writer #2:* When she went [ADV] inside to tell [INF] his dad about it, he didn't believe [MC] it either until he came [ADV] outside and saw [ADV] the broken tent and deer prints. (28 words)

In these examples, Writer #1's sentence contains only one level of hierarchical complexity, in which an infinitive clause modifies the main clause. In contrast, Writer #2's sentence contains two levels of hierarchical complexity, in which an infinitive is embedded into an adverbial clause that, in turn, modifies the main clause. Because the use of subordination and hierarchical complexity is characteristic of more advanced syntactic development, it is important to consider not only sentence length (MLTU), but also clausal density (CD) and the levels of hierarchical complexity that occur in an essay.

EXPOSITORY DISCOURSE

Spoken Language

Compared with conversational and narrative discourse, expository discourse elicits longer and syntactically more complex utterances as the speaker calls upon specialized knowledge to explain a complicated topic

TABLE 5–8. Narrative Essays Written by Two Boys with Typical Language Development (from the Author's Files)

Each essay has been coded for clause types. Note: TTU = total T-units; MLTU = mean length of T-unit; CD = clausal density; MC = main clause; NOM = nominal clause; ADV = adverbial clause; REL = relative clause; INF = infinitive clause; PRT = participial clause; GER = gerundive clause.

Writer #1: Boy, Age 11; 7 (TTU = 11; MLTU = 12.18; CD = 1.73)

One day at the mall, me and my friend went [MC] to the Home Town Buffet.

I towered [MC] three to four plates of food, one dessert plate, and two sundaes.

On the other hand, my friend had [MC] very little.

Little did I know [MC] that we had [NOM] to walk [INF] all over in the mall.

So every time I saw [ADV] a bench, I would lay [MC] down for as long as I could [ADV].

Then we went [MC] to Harry Ritchie's, Game Crazy, Radio Shack, Target, and to another video game store.

My stomach was aching [MC] the whole time.

Me and my friend both agreed [MC] I ate [NOM] way too much.

Then we had [MC] to walk [INF] way down and around the whole outside of the whole huge mall.

Then we went [MC] to the other mall and walked [MC] around.

I learned [MC] never to eat [INF] that much again.

Writer #2: Boy, Age 13; 8 (TTU = 12; MLTU = 12.58; CD = 2.42)

It all started [MC] when I went [ADV] to my friend's house to spend [INF] the night.

We set [MC] up a tent to sleep [INF] in.

Jim and I were playing [MC] games when we heard [ADV] something.

And the next thing we know [REL], a deer fell [MC] on his tent in the backyard.

It was [MC] pretty freaky.

We tried [MC] to kick [INF] him off the tent.

But it just kept [MC] moving [GER] around.

In the end, it got [MC] up and ran [MC] off back into the woods.

When we went [ADV] inside to tell [INF] his mom about it, she did not believe [MC] it at first because it was [ADV] pretty unbelievable.

But when she came [ADV] outside and saw [ADV] the broken tent and deer prints, she believed [MC] us.

When she went [ADV] inside to tell [INF] his dad about it, he didn't believe [MC] it either until he came [ADV] outside and saw [ADV] the broken tent and deer prints.

All in all, it was [MC] one weird night.

(Nippold, 2007, 2009). The *Favorite Game or Sport* (FGS) task, shown in Table 5–9, has been used in studies with adolescents having typical language development (TLD), specific language impairment (SLI), nonspecific language impairment (NLI), and autism spectrum disorders (ASD) (Nippold & Hesketh, 2009; Nippold, Hesketh, Duthie, & Mansfield, 2005; Nippold, Mansfield, Billow, & Tomblin, 2008; Nippold, Moran, Mansfield, & Gillon, 2005). With this task, the adolescent is asked to name a preferred activity and to talk about it by explaining a number of key features, including the rules, goals, and strategies needed to win the activity. Because the adolescent chooses the game or sport, it is assumed that the speaker has some familiarity with it. In those studies, adolescents' performance on the FGS task was compared with their performance on a task similar to the *General Conversation* task shown in Table 5–1. The findings indicated that both tasks were sensitive to developmental growth in the production of complex syntax during adolescence. However, it also was found that the FGS task elicited longer utterances with greater amounts of subordination than did the *General Conversation* task for adolescents with TLD, SLI, and NLI. Although the conversational task did not reveal any differences between groups, the FGS task indicated that adolescents with TLD outperformed those with SLI and NLI on measures of syntactic development. This suggests that expository tasks such as the FGS could be used to gain insight into an adolescent's ability to use complex syntax in natural speaking situations. When the task was used with adolescents having ASD, it revealed a variety of difficulties in language production (see Chapter 6).

Table 5–10 contains excerpts from the samples of two 13-year-old boys during the FGS task. Both boys were explaining how to play football. The first speaker has SLI, and the second one has TLD. Both excerpts were

TABLE 5–9. The Favorite Game or Sport (FGS) Task (Nippold, Hesketh, Duthie, & Mansfield, 2005, p. 1052)

Interviewer: I am hoping to learn what people of different ages know about certain topics. There are no penalties for incorrect answers.

A. What is your favorite game or sport?

B. Why is [e.g., chess] your favorite game?

C. I'm not too familiar with the game of [chess], so I would like you to tell me all about it. For example, tell me what the goals are, and how many people may play a game. Also, tell me about the rules that players need to follow. Tell me everything you can think of about the game of [chess] so that someone who has never played before would know how to play.

D. Now I would like you to tell me what a player should do in order to win the game of [chess]. In other words, what are some key strategies that every good player should know?

TABLE 5–10. Excerpts from the Samples of Two 13-Year-Old Boys Explaining How to Play Football During the FGS Task (from the Author's Files)

Speaker #1 has SLI, and Speaker #2 has TLD. Each sample has been coded for clause types. All mazes are enclosed in parentheses. Note: TCU = total C-units; MLCU= mean length of C-unit; CD = clausal density; MC = main clause; ADV = adverbial clause; NOM = nominal clause; REL = relative clause; INF = infinitive clause; PRT = participial clause; GER = gerundive clause.

Speaker #1 (SLI): TCU = 11; MLCU = 11.00; CD = 1.73

C (OK) All you have [REL] is [MC] 11 people (on) for offense at a time.

C You only have [MC] 11 on the field at a time for your team on offense or defense.

C (um) The goal is [MC] to (run the ball) get [INF] the ball down on the other side of the field where the end zone is [REL].

C And you score [MC] six points.

C If you make [ADV] a field goal, you get [MC] one point.

C And if you go [ADV] (for two for an extra poi) for a two point conversion, you get [MC] two points.

C You kick [MC] the ball.

C If you score [ADV], you kick [MC] the ball off to the other team.

C And they run [MC] it.

C (and then you get a chance to like) There's [MC] four downs.

C And if you only get [ADV] the four downs for the first ten yards, (and) you got [MC] to (like) give [INF] the ball to the other team.

Speaker #2 (TLD): TCU = 21; MLCU = 12.10; CD = 2.29

C (OK) There are [MC] 11 people on each team (that can) that's [REL] on the field at a time.

C So there's [MC] 22 total.

C (um) Positions are [MC] quarterback who throws [REL] the ball for people to catch [INF].

C And then there's [MC] the receivers who try [REL] to catch [INF] passes.

C (um) There's [MC] a running back.

C There's [MC] actually three running backs.

C There's [MC] a running back, a tailback, and a fullback (um) who all get [REL] hand offs and try [REL] to run [INF] up field.

C And then the rest are [MC] linemen who protect [REL] the quarterback and make [REL] holes for the running backs.

C And the whole object of the game is [MC] for your offense to take [INF] the ball down the field and score [INF] a touchdown which is [REL] worth six points.

C And then after that, you kick [MC] an extra point.

continues

TABLE 5–10. *continued*

C So a touchdown, if you get [ADV] the extra point, is [MC] worth seven.

C On defense, the object is [MC] to stop [INF] the other team's offense from scoring [GER].

C You get [MC] (four tries) four downs.

C And in those four downs, you have [MC] to get [INF] ten yards.

C And you get [MC] to keep [INF] the ball.

C And so (if you don't get four downs or) if you don't make [ADV] ten yards on four downs, then you lose [MC] the ball.

C And it's [MC] the other team's ball.

C And if it's [ADV] fourth down, and you don't think [ADV] you're going [NOM] to make [INF] it, then you can punt [MC] and put [MC] the other team further in their territory.

C And some of the rules are [MC] you have [NOM] to stay [INF] on your side of the line of scrimmage until the ball's hiked [ADV].

C (um) You can't block [MC] someone from behind.

C And there's [MC] no late hits or anything like that.

---

entered into SALT and coded for main and subordinate clauses, including finite and nonfinite clauses. Although both excerpts are relatively short, there are some interesting points to consider. Speaker #1 produced about half as many C-units as Speaker #2, suggesting that his knowledge of football was less extensive. Additionally, Speaker #1 produced shorter C-units, on average, used a smaller number and variety of subordinate clauses, and was less likely to embed subordinate clauses compared with Speaker #2 who produced C-units such as, "And if it's [ADV] fourth down, and you don't think [ADV] you're going [NOM] to make [INF] it, then you can punt [MC] and put [MC] the other team further in their territory."

The *Peer Conflict Resolution* (PCR) task, shown in Table 5–11, like the FGS task, has been used in research with adolescents having TLD, SLI, NLI, and ASD (Nippold & Hesketh, 2009; Nippold et al., 2007; Nippold et al., 2009). Adapted from Selman and colleagues (1986), the task requires the adolescent to listen to a set of conflicts between young people, reflect on the underlying issues, suggest ways they might be resolved, explain why those solutions might be successful, and indicate how the characters then might feel.

This task is of interest to adolescents because they are in a developmental stage where peer interaction is of primary importance as they learn about appropriate social behavior. Peers also are a major source of emotional support for many adolescents. Because interpersonal conflicts can be challenging to resolve and may be approached from multiple perspectives,

TABLE 5–11. Peer Conflict Resolution Task (Nippold et al., 2007, p. 187)

Interviewer: People are always running into problems with others at school, at work, and at home. Everyone has to work out ways to solve these problems. I am going to read you two different stories that illustrate these types of problems. I would like you to listen carefully and be ready to tell each story back to me, in your own words. Then I will ask you some questions about the story. There are no penalties for incorrect answers. I just want to know what you think about the issues and how they should be handled.

(In presenting the task, the interviewer should use male names with male students, and female names with female students. This pattern may increase the likelihood that students would be able to relate to the characters' actions, challenges, and emotions).

Story A: "The Science Fair"

John's (Debbie's) teacher assigned him (her) to work with three other boys (girls) on a project for the science fair. The boys (girls) decided to build a model airplane that could actually fly. All of the boys (girls) except one, a boy (girl) named Bob (Melanie), worked hard on the project. Bob (Melanie) refused to do anything and just let the others do all the work. This bothered John (Debbie) very much.

Now I'd like you to tell the story back to me, in your own words. Try to tell me everything you can remember about the story . . .

Now I'd like to ask you some questions about the story:

A. What is the main problem here?
B. Why is that a problem?
C. What is a good way for John (Debbie) to deal with Bob (Melanie)?
D. Why is that a good way for John (Debbie) to deal with Bob (Melanie)?
E. What do you think will happen if John (Debbie) does that?
F. How do you think they both will feel if John (Debbie) does that?

Story B: "The Fast Food Restaurant"

Mike and Peter (Jane and Kathy) work at a fast food restaurant together. It is Mike's (Jane's) turn to work on the grill, which he (she) really likes to do, and it is Peter's (Kathy's) turn to do the garbage. Peter (Kathy) says his (her) arm is sore and asks Mike (Jane) to switch jobs with him (her), but Mike (Jane) doesn't want to lose his (her) chance on the grill.

Now I'd like you to tell the story back to me, in your own words. Try to tell me everything you can remember about the story . . .

Now I'd like to ask you some questions about the story:

A. What is the main problem here?
B. Why is that a problem?
C. What is a good way for Mike (Jane) to deal with Peter (Kathy)?
D. Why is that a good way for Mike (Jane) to deal with Peter (Kathy)?
E. What do you think will happen if Mike (Jane) does that?
F. How do you think they both will feel if Mike (Jane) does that?

the PCR task may stimulate complex thought and sophisticated reasoning as the issues are considered. Hence, the task may prompt adolescents to use complex syntax as they articulate their views.

As with the FGS task, the PCR task was sensitive to developmental growth in syntax in terms of MLCU, clausal density, and the use of nominal and relative clauses (Nippold et al., 2007). In addition, findings revealed that adolescents with TLD outperformed their peers with SLI and NLI on measures of syntactic development, which included MLCU, clausal density, and nominal clause production (Nippold et al., 2009). As with the FGS task, performance on the PCR task of adolescents with ASD yielded mixed findings (see Chapter 6).

Table 5–12 contains excerpts from the samples of two 15-year-old boys during the PCR task. Speaker #1 has SLI, and Speaker #2 has TLD. In terms of the quantitative measures, Speaker #2 outperformed Speaker #1 on all key variables: TCU, MLCU, and CD. Qualitatively, it is interesting to examine the content of their responses to the examiner's questions, with Speaker #2 showing a bit more insight into the complexity of the issues than Speaker #1, who tended to respond in a simplistic fashion. For example, in response to the question, "How do you think they both will feel if John does that?" Speaker #2 suggested that John would have mixed emotions (feeling fine but also disappointed), whereas Speaker #1 suggested that John would be happy. Speaker #2 also tended to use more sophisticated vocabulary (e.g., *confronts, decides, refuses, disappoint, displeased*) than Speaker #1 (e.g., *tell, like, happy, angry, mad*) in his responses.

TABLE 5–12. Excerpts from the Spoken Language Samples of Two 15-year-old Boys During the PCR Task (from the Author's Files)

Speaker #1 has SLI, and Speaker #2 has TLD. Each sample has been coded for clause types. All mazes are enclosed in parentheses. Note: TCU = total C-units; MLCU = mean length of C-unit; CD = clausal density; MC = main clause; ADV = adverbial clause; NOM = nominal clause; REL = relative clause; INF = infinitive clause; PRT = participial clause; GER = gerundive clause.

Speaker #1 (SLI): TCU = 10; MLCU = 10.44; CD = 2.20

E What is the main problem here?

C John didn't like [MC] what Bob was doing [NOM].

E Why is that a problem?

C Because John doesn't like [MC] when people don't help [NOM] on projects that they're assigned [REL] to.

E What is a good way for John to deal with Bob?

C Go [MC] to the teacher and tell [MC] the teacher Bob wasn't doing [NOM] it.

C And have [MC] Bob removed [PRT] from the group.

TABLE 5–12. *continued*

E What do you think will happen if John does that?

C Either Bob will get [MC] mad (and help) and tell [MC] the teacher that he'll help [NOM] more.

C (or he'll just take ou get out get taken out of the) Or he'll respect [MC] the teacher (and not get) and get taken [MC] out of that and put [MC] in a different group.

E How do you think they both will feel if John does that?

C (angry)

C (he) He'll be [MC] happy.

C John will be [MC] happy, more satisfied.

C And Bob will be [MC] angry because he's gonna [ADV] get [INF] a failed grade for not helping [GER].

Speaker #2 (TLD): TCU = 13; MLCU = 13.00; CD = 2.77

E What is the main problem here?

C Bob will not work [MC].

E Why is that a problem?

C (uh) When you have [ADV] one person unwilling [PRT] to do [INF] any work, that means [MC] your other people in the group have [NOM] to work [INF] harder and pick [INF] up the slack for him.

E What is a good way for John to deal with Bob?

C (uh) He can confront [MC] Bob and ask [MC] him to work [INF].

C And if Bob still refuses [ADV], he can go [MC] to the teacher and ask [MC] that Bob be switched [NOM] or removed [NOM].

E What do you think will happen if John does that?

C Well, if he confronts [ADV] Bob, and Bob decides [ADV] "(fine) I'll work" [NOM], Bob will work [MC], not very well, and very disgruntily.

C If he confronts [ADV] the teacher about it, the teacher will ask [MC] the other members of the group.

C And if they all (give) give [ADV] the same answer, Bob will be removed [MC] from group.

C He will either be replaced [MC].

C Or they will end [MC] up working [PRT] by themselves still.

E How do you think they both will feel if John does that?

C John will be [MC] (uh) fine with it because now he won't have [ADV] to make [INF] up for someone else's slack.

C But it will also disappoint [MC] him because he'd still have [ADV] to do [INF] more work.

C Bob will be [MC] displeased.

C He'll have [MC] to do [INF] his own project.

Written Language

To examine the development of expository discourse in written language, Nippold and Sun (2010) conducted a study in which 11-year-old children (5th grade) and 14-year-old adolescents (8th grade; $n = 40$ per group) were asked to write an expository essay in their classrooms at school. The expository essay, titled "The Nature of Friendship," asked the students to discuss friendship and its importance, activities that friends enjoy, and factors that can build or damage friendships. The students were given an outline that contained a list of points they should address as they wrote their essays. They also were given a booklet of lined paper in which to write their essays and were allowed 20 minutes to complete their work. The task is shown in Table 5–13.

TABLE 5–13. Expository Writing Task, "The Nature of Friendship" (Nippold & Sun, 2010, p. 102)

At this time, I would like you to write an essay. Please write an essay on the topic of friendship. Friendship is very important to people of all ages—children, adolescents, and adults. Most people say they enjoy spending time with their friends. They like to talk with their friends in person or on the phone and spend time together.

The following outline will help you organize your thoughts and write a strong essay. In your essay, be sure to explain the following:

1. What is friendship?
2. Why is it important to people?
3. How can friendship make life more enjoyable?
4. What kinds of things do friends like to do together?
5. How can people become good friends?
6. What kinds of actions can damage friendships?
7. How can people remain good friends over time?

Keep this list of questions in front of you as you write your essay. As you answer each question, try to write a full paragraph of your own ideas. You will have 20 minutes to complete your work. I have given you a booklet of lined paper to use in writing your essay. Please put your name, age, and grade level on the booklet.

As you do this work, use your best writing style with complete sentences and correct grammar, spelling, and punctuation. If you aren't sure how to spell a word, make your best guess. Try to write neatly, using a pen or pencil. If you make a mistake, just cross it out or use an eraser. Keep going until I ask you to stop writing.

Do you have any questions?

The title of your essay is "The Nature of Friendship."

Results showed that the 8th graders outperformed the 5th graders on total words and sentences produced and on MLTU. Table 5–14 contains examples of expository essays written by two students in the study, an 11-year-old girl (Writer #1) and a 13-year-old girl (Writer #2).

TABLE 5–14. Excerpts of Expository Essays Written by Two Girls with Typical Language Development (from the Author's Files)

Each essay has been coded for clause types. Note: TTU = total T-units; MLTU = mean length of T-unit; CD = clausal density; MC = main clause; NOM = nominal clause; ADV = adverbial clause; REL = relative clause; INF = infinitive clause; PRT = participial clause; GER = gerundive clause.

Writer #1: Girl, Age 11; 0 (TTU = 22; MLTU = 12.05; CD = 2.64)

Do you know [MC] what friendship is [NOM]?

I do [MC].

So let [MC] me tell [INF] you.

Friendship is [MC] something you have [REL] between someone, someone you can trust [REL] and rely [REL] on.

They should be [MC] nice and thoughtful.

Also, they should never do [MC] mean or bad things to you or others.

It is [MC] important to people because you have [ADV] someone you can let [REL] something out to.

Plus they feel [MC] they have [NOM] someone always there for them.

Maybe also because then if they get [ADV] picked on, they have [MC] someone to have [INF] to help [INF] them out.

And it is [MC] fun to have [INF] friendship.

Friendship can make [MC] your life more enjoyable because you have [ADV] someone to laugh [INF] with and play [INF] with.

You can have [MC] at least someone to talk [INF] to and listen [INF] to.

When you have [ADV] a friend, you can do [MC] a lot of things like go [NOM] to the mall, in addition play [NOM] board games.

They also like [MC] to just hang [INF] out with each other.

You can become [MC] a good friend by not yelling [GER] at people and using [GER] bad words because that makes [ADV] people think [NOM] you are [NOM] a bad person.

continues

TABLE 5–14. *continued*

People will find [MC] out that you are [NOM] like that.

And nobody will want [MC] to be [INF] your friend.

Also you never want [MC] to lie [INF].

Or people won't trust [MC] you.

A lot of things can ruin [MC] your friendship like telling [GER] people their private things like family history, who they like [NOM], what they don't like [NOM] about people, and telling [GER] about embarrassing moments.

Also if someone moves [ADV] or leaves [ADV] for awhile, get [MC] their email address or phone number.

I hope [MC] your friendship lasts [NOM] a long time.

Writer #2: Girl, Age 13; 10 (TTU = 15; MLTU = 16.47; CD = 3.87)

Friendship is [MC] a strong bond between two or more people.

It is [MC] important to people because it is [ADV] someone they can talk [REL] to, hang [REL] out with, or share [REL] secrets.

Friendship is [MC] an important part of life.

It makes [MC] life more enjoyable because you are [ADV] not depressed all the time and sad and lonely.

They make [MC] life more fun.

Best friends usually hang [MC] out together, sometimes go [MC] to the mall, watch [MC] a movie, stay [MC] the night at each other's house, share [MC] their problems, and give [MC] advice.

They pretty much do [MC] everything together.

Becoming [GER] someone's best friend includes [MC] earning [GER] trust, honesty, being [GER] nice.

Most friends have [MC] a lot in common or share [MC] the same interests.

The type of actions that can damage [REL] friendships are [MC] like backstabbing [GER] most of the time, lying [GER], or being [GER] rude, fighting [GER] in most girls' friendships, fighting [GER] over boys, and who likes [NOM] who.

Stealing [GER] your friend's stuff could ruin [MC] a friendship.

Keeping [GER] a friendship and making [GER] it last a lifetime means [MC] being [GER] trustworthy, being [GER] honest, sharing [GER] your problems, trying [GER] not to fight [INF] with them or make [INF] them mad at you.

If you think [ADV] you two have [NOM] a problem and no one is trying [NOM] to work [INF] it out, just ignoring [GER] it, then try [MC] to talk [INF] to them about it and be [MC] open, help [MC] them with their problems, and help [MC] them through life, helping [PRT] make [INF] important decisions.

Just always be [MC] there for them all the time by their side all day every day.

That is [MC] what friendship is [NOM] all about, right?

Both MLTU and CD are substantially higher in the older girl's essay. The longest sentence in each girl's essay is shown here:

> *Writer #1:* A lot of things can ruin [MC] your friendship like telling [GER] people their private things like family history, who they like [NOM], what they don't like [NOM] about people, and telling [GER] about embarrassing moments.

> *Writer #2:* If you think [ADV] you two have [NOM] a problem and no one is trying [NOM] to work [INF] it out, just ignoring [GER] it, then try [MC] to talk [INF] to them about it and be [MC] open, help [MC] them with their problems, and help [MC] them through life, helping [PRT] make [INF] important decisions.

The sentence produced by Writer #1 contains four subordinate clauses, and each modifies the main clause; no subordinate clauses in this sentence are embedded within other subordinate clauses. Hence, there is only one level of hierarchical complexity. In contrast, the sentence produced by Writer #2 contains four coordinated main clauses, eight subordinate clauses, and three levels of hierarchical complexity where subordinate clauses that modify main clauses are themselves modified by other subordinate clauses.

PERSUASIVE DISCOURSE

In a developmental study, Nippold, Ward-Lonergan, and Fanning (2005) examined the ability of children, adolescents, and adults to write a persuasive essay on the controversial topic of training animals to perform in circuses. Mean ages of the three groups, respectively, were 11, 17, and 24 years ($n = 60$ per group). The task that was employed in their study is shown in Table 5–15.

Each participant was allowed 20 minutes to complete the essay. Each handwritten essay was subsequently typed and entered into SALT and coded for selected aspects of syntactic, semantic, and pragmatic development.

The results of the study indicated age-related improvements in language productivity (essay length); syntactic development (MLTU and relative clause production); and lexical development as measured by the use of adverbial conjuncts (e.g., however, finally, in conclusion), abstract nouns (e.g., realization, essence, kindness), and metacognitive verbs (e.g., realize, assess, determine). In terms of pragmatics, an age-related increase occurred in the participants' ability to consider multiple points of view in their essays. Whereas children were more likely to view the conflict from only one perspective, either favoring or rejecting the circus, adolescents and adults were more likely to consider multiple perspectives. Examples of essays written by three participants in this study—a child, an adolescent,

TABLE 5–15. Persuasive Writing Task, "The Circus Controversy" (Nippold, Ward- Lonergan, & Fanning, 2005, p. 129)

People have different views on animals performing in circuses. For example, some people think it is a **great idea** because it provides lots of entertainment for the public. Also, it gives parents and children something to do together, and the people who train the animals can make some money. However, other people think having animals in circuses is a **bad idea** because the animals are often locked in small cages and are not fed well. They also believe it is cruel to force a dog, tiger, or elephant to perform certain tricks that might be dangerous.

I am interested in learning what **you** think about this controversy and whether or not **you** think circuses with trained animals should be allowed to perform for the public. I would like you to spend the next 20 minutes writing an essay. Tell me exactly what you think about the controversy. Give me lots of good reasons for your opinion.

Please do your own work and don't share ideas with your neighbors. Be sure to double space your essay. Also, please use your best writing style, with correct grammar and spelling, and good handwriting. If you aren't sure how to spell a word, just take a guess. Do you have any questions?

---

and an adult—are presented in Table 5–16. In each essay, the use of three types of literate words has been highlighted.

In this study, writers of all ages showed interest in the task, and many expressed their views about the treatment of circus animals passionately. This pattern, coupled with the finding that the task was sensitive to developmental gains in syntax, semantics, and pragmatics, suggests that it is a useful tool for examining the ability of adolescents to write persuasive essays. After an adolescent has completed an essay, the speech-language pathologist may wish to analyze it syntactically, semantically, and pragmatically, as described in Nippold et al. (2005).

CONCLUSIONS

When evaluating the language skills of adolescents, speech-language pathologists should feel free to modify the language-sampling tasks presented in this chapter and to design new ones to examine spoken and written discourse in natural settings, such as at school where adolescents are expected to write essays or make speeches and give other formal presentations, or on the job where they are expected to explain complex matters. In designing language-sampling tasks, it is wise to remember that adolescents are more likely to use complex syntax when they are knowledgeable about the topic, interested in it, and motivated to talk or write about it.

TABLE 5–16. Persuasive Essays Produced by Participants in the Study by Nippold, Ward-Lonergan, and Fanning (2005) Study

These examples (from the author's files) were analyzed by Fanning (2004), who coded instances of three types of literate words: adverbial conjuncts [AC], metacognitive verbs [MCV], and abstract nouns [ABN]. The code follows each word (in bold).

Boy, Age 11 Years

I **think** [MCV] it is a bad **idea** [ABN] to have animals in the circus because animals should be free to do what they **want** [MCV].

They're stuck in small cages.

So [AC] there is barely enough room to get their adequate exercise.

People don't **like** [MCV] to be imprisoned.

So [AC] we should let them go.

Then [AC] they won't be forced to do tricks.

I **think** [MCV] it is cruel to train animals to do a trick because if they don't do it right, the trainers will hit them.

These are the **reasons** [ABN] why I **think** [MCV] circuses should not be allowed.

For the animals' **sake** [ABN].

Boy, Age 17 Years

A common **controversy** [ABN] is often whether or not circuses are good or bad for the **community** [ABN].

I **like** [MCV] the clowns because often times they are also animal trainers.

However [AC], there is a **downside** [ABN] to all these beneficial **factors** [ABN].

Frequently [AC], the animals are underfed and are kept in small cages.

This alone **infuriates** [MCV] animal enthusiasts everywhere.

Circuses can be cruel to animals.

Therefore [AC], they should be closed down.

If animals **feel** [MCV] threatened, they could be dangerous when they fight back.

What I **believe** [MCV] is that a circus could hire more people and have them go to clown school.

Everybody **likes** [MCV] clowns, right?

The hardest **part** [ABN] of this would be training all those clowns.

Still [AC], with a little **creativity** [ABN] and some **ingenuity** [ABN] I **think** [MCV] a clown school could be possible.

Overall [AC], I **think** [MCV] animals should not be in circuses.

continues

TABLE 5–16. *continued*

Man, Age 24 Years

A trip to the circus can be an exciting **event** [ABN] for both children and adults. The circus is a place where kids can see and almost touch their favorite wild and exotic animals.

Otherwise [AC] kids may only see the animals in books or on television.

I am not entirely against animals performing in a circus.

In addition [AC], I **believe** [MCV] there should be strict **regulations** [ABN] about proper humane **care** [ABN] for animals.

Adults tend to **perceive** [MCV] the circus through more critical eyes, **analyzing** [MCV] every trick, **assessing** [MCV] the **status** [ABN] of animals, or the **behavior** [ABN] of clowns.

Obviously [AC], there is a **dispute** [ABN] about animal **cruelty** [ABN] in **terms** [ABN] of the traveling caravan thus bringing the circus from the **heights** [ABN] of magical **essence** [ABN] to the **pits** [ABN] of **criticism** [ABN].

Sadly [AC], this **issue** [ABN] may continue for a long time to come.

In addition, the task should be cognitively challenging. For example, expository tasks that request the adolescent to explain relatively simple procedures (e.g., how to make a sandwich, how to use a hairdryer) are unlikely to reveal their ability to use complex syntax and literate vocabulary. Because language sampling with adolescents is a relatively new area of research, it is expected that new tasks will be designed, tested through research, and administered to adolescents of different age groups, ethnic backgrounds, socioeconomic levels, and geographic locations, so that normative databases can be established and used by speech-language pathologists.

CHAPTER 6

Adolescents with Autism Spectrum Disorders

*I*n this chapter, language sampling is discussed in relation to adolescents who have been diagnosed with autism spectrum disorders (ASD). This is a condition that refers to a set of developmental disabilities characterized by severe and pervasive deficits in communication and social interaction, accompanied by restricted, repetitive, and ritualistic behaviors (Nelson, 2010). In schools today, speech-language pathologists play a central role in the diagnosis, assessment, and treatment of communication disorders in students with ASD whose numbers continue to increase. Because ASD is a lifelong condition, speech-language pathologists are expected to address the communication needs of students with ASD at all educational levels. Nevertheless, given the behavioral challenges of these students, it can be difficult to evaluate their language skills and to obtain useful information during formal testing sessions. Thus, an entire chapter is devoted to this topic. To illustrate some of the challenges and how they could be met, a study is described that examined syntactic complexity in adolescents with ASD, using language sampling tasks.

LANGUAGE DEVELOPMENT IN STUDENTS WITH ASD

Children and adolescents with ASD are heterogeneous in their language and cognitive development (Howlin, 2005; Loveland & Tunali-Kotoski, 2005; Sigman & McGovern, 2005; Tager-Flusberg, 2004). Although many of them are delayed in these areas, others perform above average, and others fall somewhere in between (Baron-Cohen et al., 2005). Despite this variability, it is common for students with ASD to have deficits in language development (Tager-Flusberg, 2004). For example, they often have difficulty comprehending directions, explanations, and nonliteral forms of language such as sarcasm, jokes, idioms, and metaphors (Paul, 2007). Problems in verbal expression may include articulation errors, stereotypic phrases, echolalia, neologisms, unusual intonational and prosodic patterns, and the failure to employ certain types of words such as mental state verbs (e.g., know, think, believe; Shea & Mesibov, 2005; Tager-Flusberg, Paul, & Lord, 2005). Difficulties with narrative discourse also occur, especially in their ability to understand and explain the emotions and mental states of characters in a story (Loveland & Tunali-Kotoski, 2005).

Although students with ASD often show improvements in their receptive and expressive language abilities as they mature, the majority experience lifelong deficits in communication (Howlin, 2005; Tager-Flusberg et al., 2005). Indeed, a hallmark of ASD is the existence of serious deficits in pragmatics, the social use of language (Geurts & Embrechts, 2008; Paul, Orlovski, Marcinko, & Volkmar, 2009; Volden et al., 2009). For example, for some students with ASD who engage in conversations, social communication deficits may be evidenced in their failure to follow conventional rules of politeness such as taking turns, making topic-relevant comments, shifting topics gracefully, sharing the conversational floor (Tager-Flusberg et al., 2005), and responding to others with appropriate amounts of information (Paul et al., 2009). They also may show an obsessive focus on a narrow range of topics (e.g., city bus routes, baseball statistics) during conversations with others, along with the production of inappropriate comments or questions (Loveland & Tunali-Kotoski, 2005) and unusual vocal patterns in their speech (Paul et al., 2009).

Some students with ASD also experience deficits in specific domains of language such as syntax, the structural foundation of sentences (Bennett et al., 2008; Landa & Goldberg, 2005; Lewis et al., 2007). Although standardized tests often are used to identify syntactic deficits in children and adolescents with ASD, these tests do not necessarily indicate how a speaker uses syntax to communicate in natural speaking situations. To obtain this type of functional information, it is necessary to elicit language samples.

A STUDY OF SYNTACTIC DEVELOPMENT

To learn more about syntactic development in speakers with ASD, we conducted a small, exploratory study (Nippold & Hesketh, 2009) in which we elicited conversational and expository language samples from young adolescents who had received an educational diagnosis of ASD from their school district ($n = 4$; mean age = 12;3; age range = 10;0–14;3). Based on the report of a school-based speech-language pathologist, degrees of autism included mild ($n = 2$), mild-moderate ($n = 1$), and moderate-severe ($n = 1$). Each speaker with ASD was matched individually to a speaker with typical language development (TLD) ($n = 4$; mean age = 12;7; age range = 10;11–14;1) on the basis of chronological age and gender. According to their teachers, all students in the TLD group were free of any known disorders of language, learning, or cognition and were making acceptable progress in school. There were 2 boys and 2 girls in each group. All students in the study spoke Standard American English as their primary language, and were attending schools in western Oregon (United States). Before any testing took place, the parents of each student had signed a consent form, giving formal permission for their son or daughter to participate in the study. In addition, each participant had signed an individual assent form, indicating his or her own agreement to perform the tasks.

Tasks

Each participant was interviewed by a trained graduate student at school or at the University of Oregon Speech-Language-Hearing Center. Each interview began with a general conversation (CON) about common topics such as family, pets, and school. Following the conversation, two expository tasks were administered, the Favorite Game or Sport (FGS) task and the Peer Conflict Resolution (PCR) task. All three tasks are described in Chapter 5. When the PCR task was presented to students with ASD, pictures of the main characters accompanied each story. It was decided that pictures might increase their attention to the task, given their autistic behaviors. However, when the task was presented to students with TLD, the pictures were not used as they did not appear to be necessary to maintain their attention.

Transcription, Coding, and Analysis

Each sample (CON, FGS, and PCR) was transcribed into its own SALT file (Miller & Chapman, 2003), segmented into communication units (C-units), and coded for main and subordinate clauses. A C-unit consists of a main clause and optionally may contain one or more subordinate clauses. The sentence, Mike enjoys flipping burgers even though it gets hot in the kitchen, is a 12-word C-unit that consists of a main clause (Mike enjoys flipping burgers) and one adverbial clause (even though it gets hot in the kitchen) that is linked to the main clause. Any utterances that were less than a C-unit in that they did not contain a subject or a predicate (i.e., fragments) were placed within parentheses and excluded from analyses. All mazes (e.g., false starts, repetitions) were also parenthesized and ignored for purposes of this study. All C-units were examined for the presence of three types of subordinate clauses: relative, adverbial, and nominal. Only clauses that contained finite verbs were coded, a procedure that had been employed in previous research using the same tasks (Nippold et al., 2005, 2008, 2009). After each sample had been coded for main and subordinate clauses, clausal density was determined by summing the total number of main and subordinate clauses and dividing this sum by the total number of C-units produced. The total number of C-units served as a measure of language productivity, while mean length of C-unit (MLCU) and clausal density served as measures of syntactic complexity. All samples were coded for main and subordinate clauses by one investigator (MN) and rechecked by the other investigator (LH). The initial agreement level for the coding of all clauses was 99%. All disagreements were resolved through discussion, resulting in 100% agreement.

Results

The performance of each speaker with ASD (A) and the matched peer with TLD (T) is reported in Tables 6–1, 6–2, and 6–3, respectively, for the CON, FGS, and PCR tasks. Thus, in each table, there are four pairs of speakers: A1-T1; A2-T2; A3-T3; A4-T4. Variables of interest include Total C-units, a measure of language productivity; and Mean Length of C-unit, Clausal Density, and Relative, Adverbial, and Nominal Clause Use, measures of syntactic development in school-age children and adolescents (Nippold et al., 2005, 2007).

TABLE 6–1. Performance of Individual Speakers in the ASD (A) and TLD (T) groups on the General Conversation Task

	A1	T1	A2	T2	A3	T3	A4	T4
Total C-units	020	033	042	042	047	066	047	027
Mean Length of C-unit	05.75	06.73	08.19	06.29	08.60	05.85	06.98	07.67
Clausal Density	01.10	01.12	01.21	01.19	01.36	01.09	01.23	01.44
Relative Clause Use*	00.00	00.09	00.10	00.07	00.15	00.00	00.00	00.11
Adverbial Clause Use*	00.05	00.00	00.05	00.05	00.00	00.00	00.09	00.26
Nominal Clause Use*	00.05	00.03	00.07	00.07	00.21	00.09	00.15	00.07

*Reported as percent of C-units per sample.

TABLE 6–2. Performance of Individual Speakers in the ASD (A) and TLD (T) Groups on the Favorite Game or Sport Task

	A1	T1	A2	T2	A3	T3	A4	T4
Total C-units	023	031	108	085	078	073	032	037
Mean Length of C-unit	04.83	09.74	12.21	09.76	07.21	09.60	10.16	11.00
Clausal Density	01.00	01.55	01.77	01.49	01.23	01.55	01.34	01.76
Relative Clause Use*	00.00	00.10	00.17	00.04	00.05	00.07	00.00	00.11
Adverbial Clause Use*	00.00	00.29	00.40	00.33	00.04	00.25	00.16	00.38
Nominal Clause Use*	00.00	00.16	00.20	00.13	00.14	00.23	00.19	00.27

*Reported as percent of C-units per sample.

TABLE 6–3. Performance of Individual Speakers in the ASD (A) and TLD (T) Groups on the Peer Conflict Resolution Task

	A1	T1	A2	T2	A3	T3	A4	T4
Total C-units	028	031	048	049	069	022	053	051
Mean Length of C-unit	05.39	10.45	11.27	11.92	07.10	11.00	11.68	10.02
Clausal Density	01.07	01.61	01.56	02.02	01.14	01.45	01.43	01.53
Relative Clause Use*	00.00	00.19	00.02	00.08	00.03	00.05	00.06	00.04
Adverbial Clause Use*	00.04	00.26	00.25	00.33	00.07	00.23	00.13	00.18
Nominal Clause Use*	04	00.16	00.29	00.61	00.04	00.18	00.25	00.31

*Reported as percent of C-units per sample.

Individual Differences

Because of the small number of participants in the study, the data were analyzed informally rather than with traditional statistical tests. Below, the performance of each speaker with ASD is compared with the performance of the matched peer with TLD in terms of syntactic complexity and language productivity. These comparisons allow for a detailed analysis of each speaker, providing naturalistic information about language development. They also provide information about the effectiveness of the tasks and how, in some cases, they needed to be modified. In addition, the analyses offer some clinical implications. Thus, for each speaker with ASD, areas that might be targeted during intervention are listed.

Pair #1

A1, a 14-year-old boy with moderate to severe autism, willingly participated in the activities, evidenced by his efforts to comply with the examiner's requests throughout the interview. However, his utterances frequently consisted of fragments that did not meet the criteria for complete C-units. Of his total utterances, 67% were fragments in the CON task, 66% were fragments in the FGS task, and 64% were fragments in the PCR task. Hence, his total number of C-units, a measure of language productivity, was lower than that of T1, his matched peer, particularly on the CON and FGS tasks. In addition, many of his utterances contained grammatical errors (e.g., "Batgirl never to talk," "A lots of bugs," "Wearing the glasses black one"), and his MLCU for all three tasks (5.75, 4.83, and 5.39, respectively) was shorter than would be expected for his age (Nippold et al., 2005, 2007). Throughout the tasks, A1 produced no relative clauses and few adverbial or nominal clauses, and the restricted use of subordination resulted in low clausal density scores (CON = 1.10; FGS = 1.00; PCR = 1.07). Unfortunately, he did not increase the complexity of his utterances as he moved from conversational to expository discourse, which is in marked contrast to the expected pattern for a speaker his age (Nippold et al., 2005). These behaviors in a 14-year-old boy indicate a significant delay in syntactic development (Nippold et al., 2005, 2007), and are consistent with research linking syntactic deficits with more severe autism (Bennett et al., 2008).

Regarding the content of his discourse, many of his responses suggested that he did not understand the examiner's prompts or was unable to formulate appropriate replies. For example, during the FGS task, when asked to explain some strategies needed to win a Batman game, the activity he indicated was his favorite, he replied as follows:

> I win. A lot of fun. I win. I beat Mister Freeze. I looked at Victor. Got scared first . . . My chase after the Poison Ivy with Weiner car. I shoot it. The Great Monster. Insider the hide. I came to see Poison Ivy. What do you know?

During the PCR task, A1 was unable to retell either of the stories, so the examiner modified the task by pointing to the pictures, rephrasing parts of the stories, and asking simpler questions. This spontaneous scaffolding resulted in the production of utterances that bore at least some relevance to the situation. For example, during the Fast-Food scenario, when asked to explain the problem between Mike and Peter, A1 replied:

> Mike can't get to work there. Mike did not work the grill. Mike is leaving again. Ouch! That feels bad. He breaks it. French fries. That does taste good.

Then, when asked how Mike might help solve the problem with Peter's arm, he replied:

> Mike cannot help his arm. It cannot be fixed. He looks so scared. He must not help him. I can't help his arm. Mike's arm is broken again. He must go.

In sum, this boy required a great deal of patience, flexibility, support, and positive reinforcement from the examiner in order to perform the tasks at a basic level. Had the examiner been unwilling to deviate from the scripted activity, A1's ability to achieve at least some degree of success with the three tasks would not have been revealed.

The contrast with A1's matched typical peer, T1, also a 14-year-old boy, was striking. As reported in Tables 6–1, 6–2, and 6–3, T1's MLCU was consistently greater than A1's on all three tasks (CON = 6.73; FGS = 9.74; PCR = 10.45), as were his clausal density scores (CON = 1.42; FGS = 2.03; PCR = 2.35), reflecting the use of relative, adverbial, and nominal clauses. The tables also indicate that his syntactic complexity increased as he moved from conversational to expository discourse, with MLCU and clausal density scores higher on FGS and PCR than on CON, a pattern that is found in typically developing speakers his age. He also produced more C-units than A1, particularly on the CON and FGS tasks. Consistent with this pattern, T1 readily replied to the examiner's questions and prompts, supplying topic-relevant comments that were grammatically correct, complete, and to the point. For example, when asked to explain how to win a basketball game, T1 replied as follows:

> Usually I don't let them pass me. I try and stay on their butt so that they either go around me or stay where they're at. So I just pretty much stay put there and keep them from getting the ball. Offense is when you have the ball.

Behaviors to Target with A1

Inspection of T1's performance on the three speaking tasks offers guidance concerning the level of functional communication that can be expected of a 14-year-old boy. By comparison, A1's performance on the tasks indicated a severe deficit in syntactic development, marked by fragments, grammatical errors, and little use of subordination. A1 also showed difficulty answering questions with topic-relevant comments. The information obtained from

A1's conversational and expository samples suggests that it would be useful to target the following behaviors during language intervention:

1. Increase the production of complete and grammatically correct sentences during natural speaking situations of conversational and expository discourse.

2. Increase the production of complex sentences in spoken language through the use of relative, adverbial, and nominal subordinate clauses.

3. Increase the production of topic-relevant comments in response to questions concerning favorite activities and stories that involve peer conflicts.

Pair #2

Standing in marked contrast with A1, A2, a 13-year-old boy with mild autism, was one of the most talkative participants in the study, particularly during the FGS task where he produced 108 C-units while explaining the game of Pokémon. Although his language productivity on this task exceeded that of his matched peer, his productivity on the other two tasks, CON and PCR, was nearly identical to that of his peer. It was also found that A2's syntactic development was appropriate for his age on all three tasks (see Tables 6–1, 6–2, and 6–3) in terms of MLCU, clausal density, and the use of different types of subordinate clauses. He also employed greater syntactic complexity in expository discourse than in conversational, reflecting a pattern found in typically developing speakers of all ages (Nippold et al., 2005). For example, his ability to produce complex sentences containing multiple adverbial clauses was displayed in the following utterance during the FGS:

> Like your status, if you have really bad status or your status is very low or if your defense is very low but your attack is very high, I would recommend getting a high physical attack or something to raise your defense or protect you from really powerful attacks.

Regarding the content of his discourse, he generally responded to the examiner's prompts with topic-relevant comments. Nevertheless, he tended to provide an excessive amount of detail, particularly during the FGS task, and he often used terminology that was specific to the game (e.g., "You either choose a grass, a fire, or a water depending on which one you want best") without defining those terms. Although it was often difficult to follow his explanations because of this pattern, he proceeded as if the listener understood his comments and shared his background knowledge, suggesting a problem with perspective taking. For example, when asked to explain some key strategies about Pokémon that every good player should know, he replied as follows:

> A key strategy someone should know is the rule of elements, accuracy, and power moves, what each move does and how it may affect one player and another. Some of the moves affect three players. Some only affect two. It varies. There's a thing called a double battle. It's where you and an ally versus two other players. And you don't want to hurt your ally because who knows how much life points it has. Because you need to use something if they're both grass and you're a fire type. I would suggest finding a move that takes two of them out at once, like a move called heat wave.

As with A1, the interview with A2 required patience, flexibility, and a positive attitude from the examiner. But unlike A1, A2 was a loquacious speaker who needed little prompting to produce long and complex explanations of a topic he knew well. However, he did not appear to focus on the needs of the listener when his message was unclear.

Regarding the PCR task, A2 retold both scenarios appropriately and provided relevant responses when asked to explain the nature of the problem in each situation and how it might be resolved. It is possible that the greater structure offered by the PCR task, with its brief scenarios and focused questions, assisted A2 to organize his thoughts and speak more coherently than during the FGS task. However, there was a tendency for him to focus on the perspective of only one of the characters in each story. For example, regarding the Science Fair scenario, he explained that the main problem was that Bob was going to "get in trouble," "miss out on the assignment," or "have to do it again," without commenting on the implications of the conflict for the other members of the group.

A2's matched typical peer, T2, also a 13-year-old boy, produced levels of syntactic complexity that were slightly lower than A2's scores for MLCU and clausal density on the CON and FGS tasks (see Tables 6–1 and 6–2). However, his performance equaled or slightly exceeded A2's on the PCR task (see Table 6–3). One salient difference between these two speakers was that T2 replied to the examiner's prompts with the appropriate amounts of information, addressing the main issues in a coherent fashion, and consistently defining key terms, as when he was asked to explain the term *turnover*:

> A turnover could be like if you're dribbling down the court and somebody hits the ball away and steals it. Or if you're going up for a shot and they reject you that means they hit the ball away. That could be a turnover. A turnover could be also if you accidentally go out of bounds, the ball does, if you miss a pass or something. A turnover is a mistake that your team makes.

Another difference between these speakers was that, during the PCR task, T2 appeared to view the conflicts from multiple perspectives, expressing concern for larger issues such as the success of the project and the boys' friendship, reflecting a more mature developmental level (Selman et al., 1986). For example, with the Science Fair scenario, he explained as follows:

> The main problem I think is Bob won't work. And they need him to work to help make the project go along faster. And he won't. And it makes the other people mad which makes their group not so good . . . And it's a problem because it probably makes them not friends anymore.

Areas to Target with A2

Inspection of A2's performance on the tasks indicated that he possessed many strengths as a communicator, which included high levels of syntactic complexity and language productivity. However, in comparison with T2, he demonstrated some weaknesses that may be socially penalizing. For example, the content of his discourse was sometimes difficult to follow, particularly when he used terms that were unfamiliar to the listener, and he often appeared to be unaware of the listener's confusions during the interview. To improve the clarity of A2's discourse, while building on his strengths, it would be useful to target the following behaviors during intervention:

1. Increase his attention to the needs of the listener by training him to watch for nonverbal signs of comprehension (e.g., nodding) and confusion (e.g., frowns).

2. Increase his sensitivity to the knowledge base of others by training him to ask if his message has been understood, while using his skill with complex syntax (e.g., "Are you familiar with a strategy that is called a heat wave?").

3. Increase his ability to define key terms when discussing a topic of high personal interest by calling upon his proficiency in using relative clauses (e.g., "In the game of *Pokémon*, a heat wave is a move *that takes out two players at once*").

Pair #3

A3, an 11-year-old girl with mild to moderate autism, frequently spoke in simple utterances during each of the three tasks. Because many of her utterances were less than a complete C-unit (e.g., "everything," "brain," "too many questions"), they could not be included in the calculation of her MLCU and clausal density scores (see Tables 6–1, 6–2, and 6–3). Of her total utterances, 27% were fragments in the CON task, 14% were fragments in the FGS task, and 14% were fragments in the PCR task. Hence, on the CON task, she produced fewer C-units than her matched peer, T3. On the other two tasks, FGS and PCR, A3 produced a greater number of C-units than did T3. However, as explained below, those scores must be interpreted cautiously because the examiner deviated from the scripted interview in an attempt to respond flexibly to some challenging behaviors that A3 exhibited.

Similar to the behavior of A1, A3 did not increase the complexity of her utterances as she moved from conversational to expository discourse. Although her MLCU exceeded that of her matched peer during the CON task, she lagged behind her peer on the two expository tasks. However, during the expository tasks, she occasionally produced long, grammatically correct sentences that contained subordinate clauses, indicating that her syntax was developmentally appropriate. At one point, she stated as follows:

> I know what a lot of people my age don't. The cell is the smallest unit that has all the characteristics of life. Now if you want to know what general people my age know about games and sports, you shouldn't have picked me because I can bring a lot that I and only I know.

It was also noteworthy that, although A3 claimed to be knowledgeable of games and sports, she exhibited difficulty explaining how to play her favorite game, which she reported was *Truth or Dare*. Despite the examiner's suggestion that she choose another game to discuss, A3 protested that she did not like any games, that they were boring, and that the examiner was asking too many questions. Once the examiner agreed to stop asking questions, A3 began to talk about her interest in natural modes of transportation. At that point, with A3 in control of the interview, she produced a continuous string of 11 C-units on this topic, quite coherently, and with appropriate subordination:

> I also have a bike. But I want to expand my modes of transportation. And to go with my horse, I want a covered wagon. And plus I always ride my bike everywhere I go. And Mama drives the horrible, smelly, stinky car. But I'm natural. And I go a different way. In fact, it's not just modes of transportation. It's not just going places where I want to be natural. I never want to see a nonnatural thing in my house. Next I might want to get a Pterodactyl.

During the PCR task, A3 listened attentively to the stories and retold each one successfully. However, when the examiner began to ask her to explain the nature of the conflict and how it could be resolved, A3 protested that she did not know ("I don't know." "I have no idea." "Does this look like I know anything?" [shrugs shoulders, turns palms upward]).

Despite the examiner's efforts to simplify the questions, A3 attempted to control the interaction by repeatedly telling the examiner to stop asking questions ("No more questions") and requesting that they talk about something different. For example, during the fast food scenario, she stated as follows:

> I want to have another story. Only can they not be people because I don't like people. And you know what? Are all the stories with girls? Are they all with people? Any other creatures? What about in any other stories? Other creatures, I said, and no people.

In sum, when asked to explain the rules of a game or to discuss interpersonal issues, A3 expressed frustration, criticized the tasks, and attempted to change the subject. However, when she was allowed to direct the interaction and to talk about topics of high personal interest, her affect improved markedly as did her communication skills.

A3's matched peer, T3, also an 11-year-old girl, used simpler syntax on the CON task than did A3 in terms of MLCU, clausal density, and subordinate clauses (see Table 6–1). However, she used higher syntactic complexity on the two expository tasks than did A3 (see Tables 6–2 and 6–3). For example, T3's MLCU was 2.39 words higher than A3's on the FGS task and 3.9 words higher than A3's on the PCR task. Although T3's syntactic complexity was lower than A3's on the CON task, her syntactic complexity increased as she moved from the conversational to the expository tasks, reflecting the expected, typical pattern in spoken discourse. Moreover, during both expository tasks, T3 readily responded to each of the examiner's prompts with detailed explanations that were organized, coherent, and relevant. For example, when asked to explain how to play the game of Monopoly, she began as follows:

> Well, first you have to choose your pieces and then find out who's going to be banker. But if you're the banker, you have to choose, are you going to play the game too and be the banker, or are you going to be the banker and not play? And then the banker has to give you two five hundreds, two fifties, two one hundreds, six ones, six tens, six fives, and six twenties. And then you roll to see who goes first. And then you can't buy anything until you go around once.

Similarly, during the PCR task, T3 provided reasonable explanations that reflected concern for everyone involved, suggesting that both conflicts could be resolved by having the characters talk to each other to find out what the other was thinking. During the Science Fair scenario, when asked to explain why that was a good strategy, T3 replied that through talking, "you can let the other person know that you really do care." Thus, her comments evidenced a developmentally mature approach to resolving conflicts (Selman et al., 1986).

Areas to Target with A3

The interview with A3 indicated that she was able to use age-appropriate syntax. However, she did so only when she could direct the conversation and select the topic. Unfortunately, her communication skills quickly broke down when she was asked to discuss a topic about which she was less knowledgeable or one that she disliked. By collaborating with A3's teacher, the speech-language pathologist could generate a list of topics that would be relevant to A3's school success (e.g., science) and potentially of interest to her (e.g., alternative methods of home heating; organic farming techniques; how recycled plastic bottles can be used to build fences and decks). The speech-language pathologist and teacher could work together to promote A3's knowledge of those and other meaningful topics, which would support her ability to talk about them. Then, in this way, language intervention could target the following behaviors:

1. Increase the number and range of topics that A3 can discuss in a positive manner, using complete sentences with complex syntax.

2. Increase the frequency of answering topic-specific questions with positive, informative replies, using complete sentences with complex syntax.

3. Increase A3's willingness to engage in conversations about topics that are new or less familiar to her but of high interest to others (including her peers).

Pair #4

A4, a 10-year-old girl with mild autism, began the conversational task hesitantly, speaking slowly and producing utterances that were less than a C-unit (e.g., "or both, oh yeah, all right, good yeah"). Gradually, she began to produce longer utterances (e.g., "Oh and also I really like to draw pictures. And now I can draw horses cantering") as the examiner remained patient and supportive. For the FGS task, A4 chose dog training as her topic. Speaking guardedly, she required multiple prompts and the rephrasing of questions by the examiner in order to continue the interaction. In addition, because dog training is not a game or a sport, it was necessary to modify the questions to suit the topic (e.g., Examiner: "What are the goals of dog training? What are you trying to get your dog to do?"). Even with these modifications, A4 tended to produce only one utterance at a time rather than a string of topic-relevant utterances, responding directly to each prompt, with little spontaneous elaboration. Thus, with frequent scaffolding from the examiner, the FGS task became a conversation rather than an expository monologue. Because the tasks were modified in this way, A4's scores for language productivity must be interpreted cautiously. Had the examiner not responded in this flexible manner, it is likely that A4 would have produced far fewer Total C-units on the CON and FGS tasks.

Nevertheless, A4's performance improved markedly during the PCR task, which she appeared to find more interesting than the FGS task. For this task, she retold each scenario accurately and completely, and did so without additional prompting from the examiner, and the suggestions she offered for resolving the conflicts were creative and sophisticated. For example, for the Science Fair scenario, she indicated that it was important for the group members to try to talk with each other as a first step, and that if that did not succeed, to bring in a facilitator to avoid making people mad or hurting their feelings. It was noteworthy also that she offered a number of spontaneous comments about the stories. During the fast food scenario, she pointed out that if the characters "needed to be in a rush to get someone's order down," then they "wouldn't have time to talk this out slowly like at school." She also discussed the importance of "sharing responsibility," explaining insightfully how "it does take a lot of work to own a restaurant."

A4's syntactic complexity increased as she moved from conversational to expository discourse, reflecting the expected pattern. It should be noted also that her syntactic complexity was higher during the PCR task than the FGS task, evidenced by her MLCU and clausal density scores (see Table 6–3). Thus it appears that the PCR task, which seemed to engage her interests more fully, helped to reveal her ability to use language in a more complex, creative, and sophisticated manner. Her performance on this task indicated that her syntactic development was appropriate, as her scores were similar to those of T4, the 10-year-old girl who served as her matched peer.

However, despite their similar scores on the PCR task, T4's overall performance differed markedly from A4's. During the conversation, T4 spoke freely about preferred activities, producing multiple utterances on the same topic (e.g., "I am kind of good at tetherball. But there's only a couple of people that I can beat. And I like playing with someone that's the same as me"). Then, for the FGS task, with little prompting, T4 chose the game of *Sorry* and proceeded to explain the details of this favorite activity in a clear, efficient, and organized fashion. For example, in one uninterrupted string of 19 C-units, she described how to set up the board, how to determine which player starts, how to use the playing pieces and cards, how to disadvantage an opponent, and how to win. Then, when asked about key strategies, she explained that, "you have to be smart," "think about the other players," and trade only with those who are "closest to your home."

Similarly, during the PCR task, T4 showed a clear understanding of what was being asked of her and a mature understanding of interpersonal issues. After retelling the scenarios, she explained the nature of each conflict and offered solutions that involved compromising, making the activities more enjoyable, not making other group members angry, and not requiring authority figures to intervene. These observations suggested that she was an insightful young lady who took responsibility for resolving interpersonal conflicts.

Goals for A4

Similar to A3, A4 demonstrated the ability to use age-appropriate syntax when she spoke about topics that interested her and about which she was knowledgeable (working in a restaurant, resolving interpersonal conflicts). However, her communication skills broke down when she was asked to talk about less familiar topics. This suggests that it would be worthwhile to expand the range of topics about which A4 can converse comfortably and fluently. As with A3, this might be accomplished by consulting with her teacher and generating a list of topics that would be interesting to her and relevant to school success (e.g., the solar system, how glaciers were formed, the life cycle of an oak tree). Language intervention then could assist her to talk about those topics in a confident and informed manner. Thus, the following behaviors could be targeted for A4:

1. Increase the range of topics she can discuss confidently, using complete sentences with complex syntax.

2. Increase the frequency of answering topic-specific questions by having A4 elaborate on her replies with multiple utterances that contain complex syntax.

3. Increase her willingness to engage in conversations about topics that are new or less familiar to her but of high interest to others (including her peers).

Discussion

In this exploratory study, syntactic development was examined in young adolescents with ASD, using language sampling tasks to elicit conversational and expository discourse. Little was known about the ability of young adolescents with ASD to employ complex syntax in natural speaking tasks, particularly during expository discourse.

The findings of the study were interpreted informally because of the small number of participants, coupled with the high degree of variability that occurred, particularly in the ASD group. Under these conditions, three of the four speakers with ASD demonstrated age-appropriate syntactic development and one speaker with ASD evidenced a severe syntactic deficit. In addition, three speakers with ASD had difficulty with the tasks, requiring the examiner to spontaneously adapt the activities by modifying the questions and providing additional prompts and supports. Nevertheless, even under modified conditions, the tasks revealed helpful information about the strengths and weaknesses of each speaker with ASD.

For example, A1, a boy with moderate to severe autism, produced a large number of fragments, and many of his utterances contained grammatical errors. Those factors, combined with a short MLCU and low clausal density scores, indicated the presence of a syntactic deficit. In addition, he did not show the expected pattern of increasing the complexity of his utterances as he moved from the conversational to the expository tasks, which suggested a restricted ability to use subordination. Similarly, A3 found the expository tasks challenging, requiring the examiner to adapt the activities in a flexible manner. Indeed, A3 was able to continue the interaction only when she could talk about topics of her own choosing, primarily in the conversational genre. Thus, her MLCU and clausal density scores did not increase as she moved through the tasks. Nevertheless, under those modified conditions, she produced developmentally appropriate, complex sentences. By remaining calm and flexible with these two speakers, the examiner obtained clinically useful information, identifying a syntactic deficit in one speaker, and ruling out such a deficit in the other. The two remaining speakers with ASD, A2 and A4, also demonstrated age-appropriate syntactic development. However, qualitative analyses of their performance indicated other unique challenges. For example, during the FGS task, A2 tended to provide excessive detail when talking about his favorite game, Pokémon, and he did not attend closely to the listener's needs when his explanations lacked coherence, suggesting a problem with perspective taking. Similarly, during the PCR task, he tended to focus on the needs of only one of the characters, ignoring all others in the story. Those sorts of observations of A2, revealed by the expository tasks, could be helpful in designing intervention to build his awareness of others' perspectives in situations where he uses expository discourse, such as at school when talking with teachers and classmates.

With A4, it was useful to observe the contrast in her behavior during the two expository tasks, with greater syntactic complexity and a more fluent speaking style exhibited during the PCR task. Moreover, she appeared to enjoy the PCR task more than the FGS task, which allowed her to demonstrate her knowledge of how to resolve peer conflicts, a topic she had learned about in school. Had only the FGS task been presented, her ability to speak in this more sophisticated manner would not have been revealed.

CONCLUSIONS

This small study examined syntactic development in young adolescents with ASD by eliciting samples of conversational and expository discourse. It was found that the speaker who exhibited the most severe autism also exhibited the poorest syntactic development. The three other speakers, who had milder autism, exhibited weaknesses in organization, coherence, and perspective taking during the tasks despite having adequate syntactic development. Although the number of participants was too small to draw generalizations, the results are consistent with a pattern in which more severe autism is linked to syntactic deficits (Bennett et al., 2008). Despite the preliminary nature of the study, the findings also suggest that examining syntactic development in adolescents with ASD using natural speaking tasks can be a fruitful clinical activity. However, it is emphasized that the language sampling tasks employed in the study needed to be modified for three of the four adolescents with ASD, requiring patience and flexibility from the examiner. Had the examiner been unwilling to make adjustments, it is likely that the levels of language productivity would have been quite low for those adolescents. Thus, the tasks were not administered to those adolescents in the way in which they had been designed, or in the way in which they had been administered to the typical peers. Nevertheless, even under modified conditions, the tasks yielded useful information about each speaker with ASD, offering practical implications for intervention.

CHAPTER 7

Intervention: Conversational and Narrative Discourse

This chapter offers suggestions for ways to build the clarity, precision, and efficiency of adolescents' language in conversational and narrative discourse. In working with adolescents, it is important to present activities that are dynamic, motivating, and relevant to their daily lives in social, academic, and vocational contexts.

CONVERSATIONAL DISCOURSE

Adolescents with language disorders often struggle to express themselves when talking with their peers, leading to frustration, embarrassment, and social rejection. These sorts of problems may occur when the adolescent is unsure of what to talk about; lacks sufficient knowledge of current events or other popular topics of conversation; uses inaccurate, vague, or overly general words; or speaks in a monotonous, redundant fashion that taxes the listener. For example, consider the following string of simple sentences:

> I went to the coast. There was a storm. The storm tore off some pieces. The pieces were on the cabin. It was loud. I was so scared.

When the same information is expressed more efficiently through the use of subordinate clauses and some well-chosen words, the story suddenly becomes more exciting:

When I went [ADV] to the coast, there was [MC] a fearsome windstorm that blew [REL] some shingles off the cabin. It caused [MC] a creepy commotion.

When adolescents learn to speak in a more engaging manner, their peers may be more inclined to listen to them and to seek them out as conversational partners.

To assess the conversational skills of an adolescent, the speech-language pathologist may wish to employ the conversational tasks described in Chapter 5, the *General Conversational* task (see Table 5–1), or an adaptation of the *Chess Conversation* task (see Table 5–3). At a basic level, adolescents must have the ability to use complex syntax, literate vocabulary, and appropriate grammar. If they are lacking these fundamental skills, language intervention must address these limitations. When they have acquired these skills, they must be prompted to use them in natural communication settings. In order to do so, however, adolescents must have information to share that is of interest to others. Thus, it is worthwhile to encourage adolescents to learn about events that are happening at school or in the community. Examples might include the upcoming football game, homecoming dance, student election, science fair, or the opening of a new restaurant or shopping mall in the local area. Being well-informed about a variety of topics, continuously adding to the knowledge base, will build the cognitive foundation needed to sustain conversations.

As adolescents practice conversing with their peers about topics of mutual interest, they should be encouraged to use complex syntax and appropriate words in order to express themselves in a way that is accurate, clear, and efficient. They also should be encouraged to use positive pragmatic behaviors that promote peer interactions. Examples include listening attentively, allowing others to speak, complimenting, asking questions, expressing feelings calmly, using humor, understanding others' beliefs and values, and ignoring unpleasant remarks (Schickedanz et al., 2001).

Table 7–1 contains a list of behaviors that adolescents who are proficient conversationalists often display, while Table 7–2 contains a list of behaviors that are sometimes seen in adolescents who have language disorders. When an adolescent's conversational skills are deficient, the speech-language pathologist can assist the student to acquire positive conversational skills by serving as a supportive scaffold. A list of possible intervention goals is contained in Table 7–3, and key features of effective intervention are listed in Table 7–4. In addition, Hoskins (1996) has written an excellent guidebook on how to build conversational skills in

TABLE 7–1. Conversational Behaviors of Adolescents with Typical Language Development

---

Adolescents who are proficient conversationalists do the following (Nippold, 2000, 2007).

As **listeners**, they:

- Allow others to speak without excessive interruptions
- Listen attentively and think about what is being said
- Understand and accept different perspectives and opinions
- Ask relevant and thoughtful questions that draw others out
- Smile, nod, and make normal eye contact
- Exercise discretion with personal information
- Remain optimistic, encouraging, and supportive of others

As **speakers**, they:

- Make relevant comments that extend the topic of conversation
- Talk about topics of general interest to others
- Stay on topic, remain organized, and speak coherently
- Allow others to ask questions, comment, and otherwise contribute
- Make smooth transitions to new or related topics
- Entertain others through humor, drama, and appropriate body language
- Avoid gossiping, swearing, and making hurtful comments

---

adolescents, focusing on syntax, the lexicon, and pragmatics. Other helpful sources of information on how to design intervention to support adolescents' conversational skills may be found in Brinton, Robinson, and Fujiki (2004) and Paul and Norbury (2012).

NARRATIVE DISCOURSE

During spoken and written narrative tasks, students with language disorders, compared with their peers with typical language development, produce shorter and simpler stories that contain more grammatical errors, fewer complex sentences, fewer literate words, and fewer references to the thoughts and feelings of the characters in those stories (Liles, 1985, 1987; Merritt & Liles, 1987; Scott & Windsor, 2000; Windsor et al., 2000).

TABLE 7–2. Conversational Behaviors of Some Adolescents Who Have Language Disorders

---

As conversationalists, *some* adolescents with language disorders *may* do the following (Brinton, Robinson, & Fujiki, 2004; Paul & Norbury, 2012; Paul et al., 2009):

- Make few topic-relevant comments
- Fail to ask the speaker questions that clarify or extend the topic
- Have little to say of interest to others
- Talk excessively about topics of high personal interest
- Pay little attention to what others are saying (poor listening skills)
- Provide too little or too much information, based on needs of listener
- Show little awareness of listener's background (knowledge, opinions, feelings)
- Respond poorly to listener's verbal and nonverbal cues (e.g., boredom, sadness, interest, empathy)
- Make hurtful, biased, or inaccurate comments about others
- Laugh inappropriately (e.g., at others' misfortunes, foibles)

TABLE 7–3. Possible Intervention Goals for Adolescents with Deficient Conversational Skills

---

During conversations with peers, the adolescent will:

- Identify topics that are of high interest to others, especially to peers
- Learn about a range of topics of general interest to others
- Make appropriate transitions to new or related topics of interest to others
- Listen closely to others in order to ask questions and make topic-relevant comments
- Ask appropriate questions at the right time
- Attend closely to verbal and nonverbal cues indicating others' mental states (e.g., boredom, sadness, interest, empathy)
- Show empathy, understanding, and concern for others in verbal and nonverbal ways, including positive tone of voice, facial expressions, and body language
- Make validating and positive comments (e.g., that compliment, agree, encourage, comfort, etc.)
- Share information that is appropriate in terms of the type and amount
- Speak in an organized and coherent fashion that others can follow

---

TABLE 7–4. Key Features of Effective Intervention for Conversational Skills (Adapted from Walker, Schwarz, & Nippold, 1994)

- The speech-language pathologist directly and systematically teaches the targeted behavior(s) through explanation, modeling, use of video clips, and role-play.

- The adolescent practices the targeted behavior(s) with peers in small group settings.

- The speech-language pathologist provides clear, specific, and corrective feedback on the adolescent's performance.

- When ready, the adolescent practices the new behavior(s) in settings beyond the treatment room (e.g., cafeteria, gymnasium, classroom, school bus, shopping mall).

- The speech-language pathologist provides feedback to the adolescent on the targeted behavior(s) in natural communication settings (e.g., through coaching, cueing, and debriefing).

- The speech-language pathologist provides tangible or social rewards for appropriate conversational behaviors.

Assessment

To assess narrative discourse in adolescents, tasks should be cognitively complex in order to bring out the students' linguistic competencies. Stories with intriguing characters, unexpected twists, and exciting endings may be more appropriate than the simple narratives that often are used with school-age children (e.g., the Frog stories), tasks that are unlikely to prompt adolescents to use complex syntax and literate vocabulary.

Written Narratives

To assess written narrative production in adolescents with language disorders, the speech-language pathologist may wish to use the task, "What Happened One Day," described in Chapter 5 (see Table 5–7). Although this task has not yet been administered to students with language disorders, research with students having typical language development, ages 10 to 17 years, indicated that it was effective in eliciting original stories that were funny, sad, or scary—narratives that contained complex syntax and literate vocabulary (Sun & Nippold, 2012). After administering the task to students with language disorders, the essays could be entered into SALT and examined for MLTU, number of sentences, clause types, and clausal density.

Spoken Narratives

To examine spoken narrative production, the speech-language pathologist may wish to use the fable retelling stories that were described in Chapter 5 (see Table 5-5). As discussed in that chapter, those particular fables were motivating and of interest to adolescents with typical language development, and successfully elicited the use of complex syntax as they retold the stories.

Additionally, the speech-language pathologist may wish to select a story from the student's curriculum in English class, such as a fable. Middle school and high school students are frequently required to read, retell, and analyze fables, many of which are credited to Aesop (ca. 620–ca. 560 BC), the Greek story-teller (Grosset & Dunlap, 1947). Fables are short stories that attempt to convey important messages about life. Often the main characters are animals whose actions reflect human characteristics. In ancient Greece, the ability to tell a good fable was a mark of distinction, and orators practiced telling fables in order to gain the respect of their peers. Although superficially simple, fables often contain complex syntax and literate vocabulary, concluding in a moral or proverb.

A fable that could be used for this purpose, *The Dog and His Shadow*, is shown in Table 7–5. Syntactically it is quite complex. For example, its final sentence, which is 25 words long, contains two participial [PRT] clauses and three relative [REL] clauses:

So saying [PRT], the greedy dog snapped [MC] at his reflection in the water, losing [PRT] the bone he had stolen [REL], which fell [REL] into the water and sank [REL].

Lexically, the fable includes difficult words (peace, reflection, greedy, substance, covet), and the listener or reader must understand the symbol-

---

TABLE 7–5. Example of a Fable to Be Used for Story Retelling (Lawrence, 1997, p. 33)

"The Dog and His Shadow"

One day a dog stole a bone from a butcher shop and was carrying it home in his mouth to eat in peace. On his way home, he had to cross a plank over a river. Upon looking down, he saw his reflection in the water.

"What a delicious bone that strange dog is carrying!" he growled to himself. "I must have it."

So saying, the greedy dog snapped at his reflection in the water, losing the bone he had stolen, which fell into the water and sank.

Moral/Proverb: "Grasp at the shadow and lose the substance," or "All covet, all lose."

---

ism in which the *shadow* (the dog's reflection) represents a false image (the perfect life, unattainable "riches," what we *think* we need), and the *substance* (the bone) represents reality (what we already have but may not realize). Understanding the symbolism leads to an appreciation of the moral, that the quest for more than we need causes a great loss. This, in turn, may prompt reflection on deeper questions such as, "*Why* do some people want more than they actually need?"

After an adolescent has retold the fable, it can be transcribed, entered into SALT, and coded for the use of subordinate clauses and literate words. Other useful data that are calculated automatically by SALT include the total number of words and utterances (sentences) produced and mean length of C-unit (MLCU). Clausal density can be calculated by adding the number of main and subordinate clauses together, and dividing this sum by the total number of C-units. Individual sentences can be analyzed for hierarchical levels as an additional measure of syntactic complexity.

Intervention

Regarding intervention, storytelling with fables is potentially a profitable route. During the cognitive stage of formal operational thought, adolescents become interested in abstract topics such as moral dilemmas that do not have obvious, clear-cut solutions. Because of the complexity of the underlying messages, fables may prompt the use of complex syntax and literate vocabulary as the adolescent retells and interprets the story. When using fables for narrative intervention, it is helpful if the stories are geared to the students' reading levels, yet are written in a relatively mature style. Numerous versions of Aesop's fables have been translated into English from Greek and are readily available in most libraries. Pictures that add intrigue and capture the attention of the reader or listener accompany many of these translations (e.g., Grosset & Dunlap, 1947).

The ability to retell a fable successfully requires, first of all, that the adolescent comprehend the story. Comprehending a fable involves tracking the sequence of events, processing complex syntax, understanding literate vocabulary, and grasping the perspectives of the characters. A hypothetical example of how to conduct intervention using fables is now described. Highlights of this approach are shown in Table 7–6.

The scenario is that two adolescents with SLI and three adolescents with NLI (ages 12–14 years; mean age = 13;7 years) are working together with the speech-language pathologist. The group meets three times a week at the middle school for 30-minute sessions. All five students have deficits in syntactic and lexical development and poor reading skills. The speech-language pathologist has made the assumption that to retell a fable successfully, a student must have a clear and detailed understanding of the story. To address both the comprehension and production of narratives,

TABLE 7–6. Highlights of an Intervention Approach for Narrative Discourse

- The speech-language pathologist works with students in small groups that meet frequently.
- Students are encouraged to support each other and to use appropriate pragmatics.
- Fables are chosen from the regular education curriculum.
- The understanding of fables is promoted to support their retelling.
- Written language is used to support spoken language.
- A graphic organizer is used for each fable, highlighting story grammar elements:
  - Setting
  - Characters
  - Problems
  - Solutions/attempts
  - Outcomes
  - Reactions
  - Ending/resolution
- Students fill in the graphic organizer before attempting to retell the fable.
- As a student retells a fable, the story is entered into a laptop computer.
- The document is saved, and changes are made as the students make progress.
- Sentence-combining activities are used to encourage complex syntax.
- Students discuss the meanings of difficult words and complex concepts.
- Students think about the meaning of the fable in relation to their own lives.

the speech-language pathologist has established the following goals for each member of the group:

Goal #1: The student will understand fables drawn from the regular classroom.

Goal #2: The student will retell fables drawn from the regular classroom by:

    A. Using a greater number of subordinate clauses

    B. Using a greater number of literate words

    C. Increasing the total number of words produced

    D. Increasing the total number of utterances produced by:

        1. Including a greater number of story grammar elements

        2. Including more references to the characters' thoughts and feelings

Strategies

To accomplish these goals, the students are encouraged to support each other and to use appropriate pragmatic behaviors (e.g., turn-taking, listening, patience, showing respect) during every session. Additionally, the speech-language pathologist uses written language as a tool to support spoken language during intervention by having the students refer to a printed copy of the fable, having them fill out a graphic organizer listing all story grammar elements, and having them create a written record of the story as they retell it.

Example #1

For their first fable, the students, in consultation with the speech-language pathologist and classroom teacher, choose "The Dog and His Shadow" (see Table 7–5). In terms of readability, this version of the fable has a Flesch-Kincaid Grade Level of 4.8 (Microsoft Word, 2007). Each student holds a printed copy of the fable, and all students listen as the speech-language pathologist reads the story aloud. The students underline any difficult words they encounter. Then they take turns reading the fable aloud, a process called repeated oral reading, which helps to build fluency and comprehension (Reutzel, 2009; Robertson, 2009). Those with more severe deficits in reading will receive additional intervention that addresses those issues. Next, the students are asked to think about any difficult words or expressions they encounter (e.g., eat in peace) and to attempt to infer the meaning of those linguistic units from the broader context.

To assist the students in retelling the fable, the speech-language pathologist gives them a graphic organizer, which is an outline that lists each story grammar element (setting, characters, problems, attempts/solutions, outcomes, inner and outer reactions, ending/resolutions). As they listen to the fable read aloud again, they attempt to fill out the outline, which provides them with an organizational structure for future retellings of the narrative.

As the students attempt to retell the fable, their sentences are typed into a laptop computer to create a running record of their narrative production. Either the students themselves (if they are able) or a scribe (a speech assistant) creates this document, which is saved and later modified as they make progress in subsequent retellings of the fable.

One student, a 13-year-old girl with NLI, begins to tell the fable as follows:

> Well, there's this dog. And, um, he stole this bone. And, uh, he was taking it home. He wanted to eat it by hisself. And, um, he had to cross a river.

The speech-language pathologist notes that this is a good start, but that the girl has used mostly simple sentences. To encourage her to use complex sentences, the speech-language pathologist decides to use sentence combining activities, knowing that this is an evidence-based approach, supported by research (Eisenberg, 2006; Graham & Perin, 2007; Saddler & Graham, 2005; Scott & Nelson, 2009). The speech-language pathologist provides a model by presenting two simple sentences and combining them into one complex sentence that contains a relative clause (REL):

> There was a dog. He stole a bone.
>
> There was a dog who stole [REL] a bone.

The speech-language pathologist briefly discusses how the revised sentence is more informative and efficient. Then, the new complex sentence is entered into the laptop, and the two simple sentences are deleted as the students observe. Next, the speech-language pathologist asks the same student to combine two additional simple sentences into one complex sentence. The speech-language pathologist prompts the girl as follows:

> The dog was taking the bone home so that . . .

The student then replies:

> He was taking it home so he could eat [ADV] it by hisself.

The speech-language pathologist notes that the girl has produced an adverbial clause (ADV). Praising her enthusiastically, the speech-language pathologist points this out to the other members of the group. The grammatical error also is addressed by asking the group for feedback (e.g., "How could we say that better?"). Then, the final corrected, complex sentence is entered into the computer, and the two simple sentences are deleted as the students watch the screen.

Moving on, the speech-language pathologist selects another student, a 12-year-old boy with NLI, to continue the story. He produces the following simple sentences:

> The dog looked down at the water. He saw another dog.
>
> But it wasn't another dog. It was a reflection of him.

The speech-language pathologist prompts the boy to combine the first two simple sentences into one complex sentence by presenting an adverbial [ADV] clause and part of a main clause [MC]:

> When the dog looked [ADV] down at the water, he thought [MC] . . .

Because the main clause in the speech-language pathologist's sentence starter contains a metacognitive verb (thought), it is likely to elicit a nominal clause. As predicted, the boy repeats the speech-language pathologist's sentence starter, and completes it with a nominal (NOM) clause:

> When the dog looked down at the water, he thought he saw another dog.

Once again, the complex sentence is entered into the computer, and the old sentences are deleted. In this way, the sentence-combining activities continue with other students in the group. Eventually, the full story is entered into the computer, and the revised document, written by the entire group using complex syntax, serves as the basis for retelling the fable. All students will have numerous opportunities to practice reading the story aloud and then retelling it, at first referring to the written document and later retelling it from memory.

Systematic Reflection

Throughout these activities, the speech-language pathologist pauses to encourage the students to think about the deeper meaning of the fable and how it might apply to their own lives. The purpose of this strategy, called *systematic reflection*, is to build their understanding of the story as a way of assisting them to retell it in a complete and meaningful way. Thus, the strategy is implemented by asking questions such as, "Have you ever met anyone like the dog?," "What did that person do?," "What was that person trying to obtain?," "Why did the person act that way?," "What happened in the end?" During these sessions, students are encouraged to think about the meanings of difficult words and to define them using the Aristotelian formula, "An *X* is a *Y* that *Z*." Research has shown that Aristotelian definitions express meaning in a clear and efficient manner, one that is valued in literate contexts (Nippold, 2007). Moreover, in using Aristotelian definitions, students are prompted to produce high-density sentences (e.g., "Greed is a state of mind in which people want [REL] more things than they need" [REL]) while building their knowledge of words, a technique that addresses both complex syntax and the literate lexicon.

Example #2

After achieving success with the first fable, the students choose another fable from the curriculum. This time, in consultation with the speech-language pathologist and classroom teacher, they choose a more challenging fable, "The Fox and the Crow," shown in Table 7–7. In terms of readability, this version of the fable has a Flesch-Kincaid grade level of 6.5 (Microsoft Word, 2007). Analysis of the story indicates a number of difficult words, including nouns (glory, flattery, caw), verbs (spied, watered, surpass), and adjectives (wily, charming, delightful, exquisite, vain, pleased,

TABLE 7–7. More Difficult Fable to Be Used for Story Retelling (Lawrence, 1997, p. 25)

"The Fox and the Crow"

A crow flew to the top of a tree to enjoy a piece of cheese she had stolen. A wily fox spied the cheese in the crow's beak, and his mouth watered for it, as he spoke these words:

"O beautiful crow, charming crow, delightful crow, how wonderful to see you in all your glory!"

The crow smiled, holding the cheese firmly in her beak.

"You are the most exquisite of birds—and though I have not heard your voice, I am quite sure it must surpass that of any other bird."

The vain crow was pleased by all this flattery, especially the part about her voice, for she had sometimes been told that her caw was unpleasant. She opened her beak to sing for the fox, and out fell the cheese into the fox's watering jaws.

Moral/Proverb: "Beware of flattery."

---

unpleasant, watering). Thus, in order for the students to understand the fable, it will be necessary to spend a sufficient amount of time supporting them as they learn the meanings of the words by attending to context clues and consulting a dictionary.

As with the first fable, each student will have a printed copy of the story and a graphic organizer containing story grammar elements. They will take turns reading the fable aloud, underlining difficult words, and discussing their meanings. Those who continue to struggle with reading will receive additional intervention to address their individual deficits. Additionally, all students will be encouraged to use Aristotelian definitions when explaining to each other the meanings of abstract nouns, a way to address both the literate lexicon and the use of relative clauses as they produce sentences such as the following:

"*Flattery* is a type of praise that is overly positive."

"*Hypocrisy* is a state where people pretend to be nice."

After filling out the graphic organizer, they will be asked to retell the story in their own words. This will be challenging because in addition to its difficult vocabulary, the fable contains some long and complex sentences, such as the following example:

The vain crow was [MC] pleased by all this flattery, especially the part about her voice, for she had sometimes been told [ADV] that her caw was [NOM] unpleasant.

As the students begin to retell the fable, their sentences will be entered into the laptop computer. Once again, they will be encouraged to combine simple sentences into complex sentences, with the speech-language pathologist serving as a supportive scaffold. To prompt the use of nominal clauses, for example, the speech-language pathologist will present sentence starters that contain later developing metacognitive verbs to elicit sentences such as the following:

The reader can *assume* that the fox was hungry.

The crow *assumed* that the fox was sincere.

The fox *assumed* that the crow was naïve.

To further assist the students to produce complex sentences, the speech-language pathologist will discuss with the group how different types of subordinate clauses can add information to a sentence. This represents a strategy of attempting to build the students' metalinguistic awareness by focusing their attention on specific words and structures, for there is evidence that metalinguistic activities can enhance the use of complex sentences in students with SLI and other language weaknesses (Hirschman, 2000). Thus, in the following examples, the speech-language pathologist will point out how the relative clause provides more information about the *subject* of the sentence:

The *fox*, who was [REL] very clever, was flattering the crow because he . . .

The *crow*, who was [REL] quite vain, opened her mouth because . . .

For the sake of contrast, the speech-language pathologist will also discuss with the students how, in the next two examples, the relative clause provides more information about the *object* of the sentence:

The fox tricked the *crow*, who was [REL] quite vain.

The crow dropped the *cheese*, which she had held [REL] tightly in her beak.

Moving on to other types of subordinate clauses, the speech-language pathologist will discuss with the students the use of left-branching adverbials (e.g., *When the crow opened [ADV] her mouth*, she dropped the cheese) contrasted with right branching adverbials (e.g., The crow dropped the cheese *when she opened [ADV] her mouth*) and nominals in subject position (e.g., *That he wanted [NOM] the cheese* was obvious) contrasted with nominals in object position (e.g., It was obvious to the reader that *the crow was [NOM] naïve.*). As before, each sentence will be visible on the computer screen throughout these discussions.

Once again, to promote a deeper level of understanding of the fable—an effort to ensure a stronger retelling of it—the speech-language pathologist will encourage the students to engage in systematic reflection. This might be accomplished by discussing the nature of concepts such as *hyperbole*, *vanity*, and *hypocrisy* and posing questions such as, "Have you ever met anyone like the fox? Has anyone ever tried to flatter you? When did that happen? What was that person trying to accomplish? What happened in the end?" Because these questions are designed to stimulate complex thought, it will be necessary to allow students time to generate the types of meaningful answers that are likely to require the use of complex language. Thus, it will be important for the speech-language pathologist to exercise patience, to listen attentively, and to allow the students to respond to the questions without interruption.

CHAPTER 8

Intervention: Expository and Persuasive Discourse

This chapter discusses two genres that call upon even higher levels of cognitive and linguistic competence than conversational or narrative discourse —expository and persuasive. Intervention that addresses adolescents' spoken and written language skills in these two genres should attempt to build success in academic and vocational endeavors.

EXPOSITORY DISCOURSE

Expository discourse, the use of language to convey information, is an essential genre because it is often called upon in school and at work as adolescents give oral reports in classes such as English, history, and social studies; describe to their teachers and classmates how to conduct a chemistry experiment; or perform a summer job in which they must speak with the public in person or on the telephone, explaining with clarity, precision, and confidence how to use a new cell phone, install an antivirus program on a laptop computer, or care for a sick or injured pet until the veterinarian is available.

Unlike the dialogic nature of conversation, expository discourse is more of a monologue in which the speaker bears the primary responsibility for successful communication. It is also heavily knowledge driven (Nippold, 2010a), and for this reason, language intervention for expository discourse should focus on academic topics, making it relevant to classroom success. Although classroom teachers are responsible for ensuring that students acquire knowledge of a particular subject, such as science, history, or mathematics, the speech-language pathologist can work closely with teachers in these classes, helping to build the knowledge base to support expository discourse. This can be accomplished by targeting meaningful classroom assignments such as upcoming speeches, reports, or other presentations in which the speech-language pathologist can promote the use of complex syntax, the literate lexicon, and appropriate pragmatics in spoken and written communication for a genuine purpose.

An example of how this might be accomplished is now described. The highlights of this approach are listed in Table 8–1. The scenario is that three 15-year-old boys with specific language impairment (SLI) have been assigned by their biology teacher to work as a group to make an oral report in class. The report will take place in about four weeks. Together, the boys choose the topic, "Life in the Grasslands." Table 8–2 presents a passage from their textbook, which will serve as a major source of information for their report. Note, however, that the passage contains many literate words that have been highlighted. In Table 8–3, the same passage is shown with the subordinate clauses highlighted. An examination of this passage suggests that it will be challenging to the boys because it

TABLE 8–1. Highlights of an Intervention Approach for Expository Discourse

- Target meaningful assignments from the classroom, for example, oral reports.
- Work with classroom teachers to build the knowledge base in a specific domain (e.g., biology) as a foundation for strong expository discourse.
- Assign students to work cooperatively in pairs or in small groups.
- Support students as they produce an expository document.
- Use laptop computers to create a running record of the document.
- Save and continuously modify the document.
- Use sentence-combining and sentence completion activities.
- Combine the literate lexicon with complex syntax:
  - Subordinate conjunctions with adverbial clauses
  - Metacognitive /metalinguistic verbs with nominal clauses
  - Aristotelian definitions with relative clauses
- Use repeated oral reading of complex sentences.
- Encourage summarization of content.
- Provide many practice sessions of oral report to build confidence.

TABLE 8–2. Reading Material for Oral Report, with Literate Words Highlighted in **Bold** (Adapted from Biggs et al., 2002, p. 83)

> Textbook Passage: "Life in the Grasslands"
> Literate Words: **Nouns, Verbs, Adjectives**

Grasslands are large **communities** covered with grasses and **similar** small plants. They occur in **climates** that **experience** a dry **season**, where **insufficient** water **exists** to **support** forests. Called **prairies** in Australia, Canada, and the United States, **grasslands** contain fewer than ten to 15 trees per **hectares**, though larger numbers of trees are found near streams and other water **sources**. This **biome occupies** more area than any other **terrestrial biome**, and it has a higher **biological diversity** than deserts, often with more than 100 **species** per acre. Because they are **ideal** for growing cereal grains such as oats, rye, and wheat, which are different **species** of grasses, **grasslands** have become known as the **breadbaskets of the world**.

Source: Biggs, A., Gregg, K., Hagins, W. C., Kapicka, C., Lundgren, L., Rillero, P., & National Geographic Society, *Biology: The Dynamics of Life*, page 83, Copyright 2002, The McGraw-Hill Companies, Inc.

TABLE 8–3. Reading Material for Oral Report, with Subordinate Clauses Highlighted in **Bold** (Adapted from Biggs et al., 2002, p. 83)

> Textbook Passage: "Life in the Grasslands"
> Subordinate Clauses: **Participial, Relative, Infinitive, Adverbial, Gerundive**

Grasslands are large communities **covered with grasses and similar small plants**. They occur in climates **that experience a dry season, where insufficient water exists to support forests. Called prairies** in Australia, Canada, and the United States, grasslands contain fewer than ten to 15 trees per hectares, **though larger numbers of trees are found near streams and other water sources**. This biome occupies more area than any other terrestrial biome, and it has a higher biological diversity than deserts, often with more than 100 species per acre. **Because they are ideal** for **growing cereal grains** such as oats, rye, and wheat, **which are different species of grasses**, grasslands have become known as the breadbaskets of the world.

Source: Biggs, A., Gregg, K., Hagins, W. C., Kapicka, C., Lundgren, L., Rillero, P., & National Geographic Society, *Biology: The Dynamics of Life*, page 83, Copyright 2002, The McGraw-Hill Companies, Inc.

places high demands on their language skills. For example, given their documented deficits in lexical and syntactic development, they can be expected to have difficulty comprehending the passage as it is read aloud to them and when they attempt to read it to themselves. The passage also assumes some background knowledge of related topics (e.g., geography, climatology, edible plants). Despite these challenges, much can be done to help the boys succeed with their oral report, particularly when the speech-language pathologist establishes reasonable goals, has a systematic plan for helping them achieve those goals, is able to work with them frequently, and maintains a positive attitude. Hence, the speech-language pathologist has established the following goals for each member of the group:

Goal #1: The student will understand passages from the biology text.

Goal #2: The student will explain the content of the passages as follows:

   A. Using a greater number of complex sentences, including

       1. Adverbial clauses

       2. Relative clauses

       3. Nominal clauses

   B. Using a greater number of words and utterances

   C. Using domain specific technical vocabulary

To begin, it is helpful if the boys have access to a laptop computer, know how to use it, and have accurate keyboarding skills. This will allow them to create a running record of their oral report, which will be written in the expository genre. If necessary, a scribe or speech assistant may be called upon to write down what the students would like to say. This document then will be saved and modified over time as the boys make improvements to it, adding information and using complex sentences and literate words.

For this group of boys, the speech-language pathologist has chosen to read short excerpts of the biology passage to them because they often become frustrated with independent reading assignments. As the speech-language pathologist reads the passage aloud, the boys follow along on their own printed copies of it. Then the boys are asked individually to retell as much of the excerpt as they can remember, in their own words. Their exact words and sentences are entered into the computer as they watch the screen. Here is what the boys have said:

Grasslands are large pieces of land.

They are covered with grasses and small plants.

Trees do not grow well in grasslands.

But sometimes trees can grow near streams or rivers.

Although this is a good start, the speech-language pathologist notes that they have produced all simple sentences. To increase their use of complex syntax, and hence the efficiency of their communication, the speech-language pathologist decides to engage the boys in some sentence-combining activities, knowing that this technique is supported by research (e.g., Eisenberg, 2006; Graham & Perin, 2007; Saddler & Graham, 2005; Scott & Nelson, 2009). The speech-language pathologist begins by modeling an example of how to do this. This is what she says:

> Trees grow well. It rains often.
>
> Trees grow well when . . . it rains often.

After presenting several more examples, the speech-language pathologist asks the boys to combine two of the simple sentences that they have written into one complex sentence. They begin with the following sentences, which appear on the screen of the laptop computer:

> Grasslands are large pieces of land.
> They are covered with grasses and small plants.

To assist the boys, the speech-language pathologist reads the first sentence aloud, pauses, and then prompts them to complete it with the second sentence by providing an appropriate relative pronoun:

> Grasslands are large pieces of land *that* . . .

This leads the boys to produce a complex sentence that contains a relative clause:

> Grasslands are large pieces of land *that are covered with grasses and small plants*.

This revised sentence then is entered into the computer, and the two simple sentences are deleted. It is interesting to note that the complex sentence that they have just produced is actually an Aristotelian definition, which follows the formula, "An *X* is a *Y* that *Z*." Aristotelian definitions constitute a clear and efficient way to express meaning, and for this reason, they frequently occur in formal communication (Nippold, Hegel, Sohlberg, & Schwarz, 1999). Moreover, the ability to produce these definitions is associated closely with academic achievement in adolescents (Nippold, 1999). Table 8–4 contains an example of an Aristotelian definition that occurred in a science textbook. It shows how multiple levels of embedding can be organized to express a great deal of information efficiently.

Next, the speech-language pathologist moves to the second set of simple sentences, which appear on the computer screen:

> Trees do not grow well in grasslands.
> But sometimes trees can grow near streams or rivers.

TABLE 8–4. Example of an Aristotelian Definition Contained in a Science Textbook (Biggs et al., 2002, p. 83)

> Aristotelian definitions commonly occur in expository passages:

Other important prairie animals include prairie dogs, which are [REL] seed-eating rodents that build [REL] underground "towns" known [PRT] to stretch across mile after mile of grassland, and the foxes and ferrets that prey [REL] on them.

Source: Biggs, A., Gregg, K., Hagins, W. C., Kapicka, C., Lundgren, L., Rillero, P., & National Geographic Society, *Biology: The Dynamics of Life*, page 83, Copyright 2002, The McGraw-Hill Companies, Inc.

Once again, the speech-language pathologist reads the first sentence aloud and then pauses. This time, however, she prompts them to complete it by providing an appropriate subordinate conjunction:

Trees do not grow well in grasslands *unless* . . .

But sometimes trees can grow near streams or rivers.

This leads them to produce a complex sentence with an adverbial clause:

Trees do not grow well in grasslands *unless they are near streams or rivers.*

As before, the new sentence is entered into the laptop, and the old sentences are deleted.

Thus far, the intervention activities have prompted the boys to produce complex sentences that contain relative and adverbial clauses. To prompt the use of nominal clauses, the speech-language pathologist decides to focus on some metacognitive (e.g., *assume*) and metalinguistic (e.g., *claim*) verbs that occur in other passages of the biology book.

The goal will be for the boys to produce complex sentences such as the following:

Biologists assume *that thousands of buffalo once roamed [NOM] the grasslands.*

Botanists claim *that some wildflowers grow [NOM] well in grasslands.*

These types of sentences might be elicited by asking specific questions, which require knowledge of the subject matter, and then offering a sentence to be completed:

Q: What do biologists assume?

A: They assume that . . .

Q: What do botanists claim?

A: They claim that . . .

As the boys make progress with this type of exercise, they can be encouraged to produce sentences that contain embedded subordinate clauses, for example:

Q: Why do botanists make that claim?

A: They make that claim *because they know [ADV] that certain flowers, such as blazing stars, are [NOM] drought-resistant.*

At each intervention session with the speech-language pathologist, the boys will add several complex sentences to the document they are writing concerning life in the grasslands, using these types of activities. As each new sentence is added, each boy will be requested to read and reread the document aloud, a technique called *repeated oral reading* that helps to build reading fluency (Reutzel, 2009; Robertson, 2009). It also provides an opportunity for the boys to practice using complex sentences in oral language. Then, after repeatedly reading the document aloud, they will each be asked to summarize, in their own words, what they have written. Over time, these oral summaries should contain greater amounts of relevant information, conveyed through an increased use of complex sentences.

After spending time on these intervention activities, the boys will need to practice delivering their oral report in order to refine their speaking abilities and build confidence. During these practice sessions, they will be allowed to refer to note cards. However, they will be expected to present their report by speaking primarily from their knowledge base, because it is their understanding of the topic that will support their use of complex syntax and literate vocabulary during expository discourse. As they practice, the speech-language pathologist will provide feedback on additional factors that will impact their delivery, such as speech rate, articulation, vocal intensity, facial expressions, and eye contact. The speech-language pathologist also will need to address any grammatical errors that occur (e.g., failure to use past irregular verb forms correctly).

In sum, activities that encourage adolescents to combine literate vocabulary (e.g., abstract nouns, subordinate conjunctions, metacognitive verbs) with complex syntax (e.g., relative clauses, adverbial clauses, nominal clauses) as they discuss the material they are learning in the classroom provide needed practice in using expository discourse in formal speaking contexts. A long-term goal is that they will be able to express themselves with greater accuracy, precision, and efficiency when speaking in the expository genre about many different topics. Given the speech-language pathologist's knowledge and appreciation of the complex nature of spoken and written communication, it is clear that this professional can make a unique contribution to the academic success of adolescents.

PERSUASIVE DISCOURSE

With persuasive discourse, a speaker or writer takes a position on a controversial topic and tries to convince other people to agree with his or her point of view (Gage, 1991). According to British philosopher Stephen Toulmin (1958), to be effective, the persuasive speaker or writer must support claims with evidence, acknowledge and rebut the opposing point of view, and draw logical conclusions based on the information presented. During childhood, adolescence, and into adulthood, performance on persuasive tasks gradually improves, with measurable growth occurring in the ability to consider both sides of an issue, to appeal to others' values and beliefs, to present multiple reasons for a particular claim, and to use complex syntax and literate vocabulary to communicate clearly and efficiently (Nippold, 2007; Nippold, Ward-Lonergan, & Fanning, 2005). However, children and adolescents with language and learning difficulties often struggle to produce persuasive discourse that is well-organized, rich in content, and addresses diverse points of view (Wong et al., 1996).

Intervention designed to build students' persuasive speaking and writing skills presents an opportunity for the speech-language pathologist to work collaboratively with classroom teachers to help students succeed academically. In schools today, it is common in classes such as science, history, and health for students to be asked to engage in debates with their classmates and to write persuasive essays, either alone or with peers, in which they must take a position and defend it with solid arguments. However, to be successful at persuasive speaking or writing, it is critical that students know something about the topic, are motivated to discuss it, and believe that their efforts will make a difference.

Thus, it is important that students be allowed to select the topic they will address and that they be encouraged to learn more about it by reading books and magazines and searching the Internet for informative articles. It is helpful also if they can work together in small groups in which different points of view can be voiced and discussed. An example of how this type of intervention might be carried out is now presented (also see Nippold & Ward-Lonergan, 2010). Table 8–5 lists the highlights of the approach.

Intervention Scenario

In an 8th-grade health class, a group of six students (two of whom have SLI) decide to debate the issue of leisure-time activities. Three of the students strongly believe that young people their age should participate in physical activities after school, such as playing basketball, tennis, and baseball, or hiking, running, and swimming. However, the other three

TABLE 8–5. Highlights of an Intervention Approach for Persuasive Discourse

---

- Speech-language pathologist works collaboratively with classroom teacher (e.g., history, science, health).

- Students work together in small groups with speech-language pathologist.

- Students in consultation with speech-language pathologist and teacher select topic to debate.

- Students are encouraged to learn more about the topic.

- Brainstorming activities occur to stimulate discussion about the topic.

- Subgroups defend own point of view and consider other side of issue.

- Reasons are offered, based on documented information.

- Points on both sides of the issue are typed into the laptop computer.

- The document is saved and modified as more information is added.

- Students are encouraged to use literate vocabulary and complex syntax.

- Students use full sentences with correct grammar and spelling.

- Students use words that are precise, accurate, and engaging.

- Students use graphic organizer to write persuasive essay:
  - State topic and explain why it is controversial.
  - State own opinion clearly (in my opinion . . .).
  - Give different reasons for own opinion (first of all, second, third, finally).
  - State what others believe (on the other hand, some people believe . . .).
  - Explain why they believe that way (they believe this because . . .).
  - Summarize own opinion and conclude the essay (nevertheless, I still believe . . . I believe this because . . . In conclusion . . .).

---

students strongly believe that after a full day of school, it is more beneficial to engage in less active pastimes such as watching television, playing video games, reading and sending e-mail, talking on the phone, or text-messaging with friends.

For the two students with SLI, the speech-language pathologist has established the following goals:

Goal #1: The student will write an essay that considers both sides of an issue.

Goal #2: The student will write an essay that is well-organized.

Goal #3: The student will write an essay that includes complex language:

A. Literate vocabulary

   1. Adverbial conjuncts (e.g., consequently, therefore, however)

   2. Metacognitive verbs (e.g., expect, assume, infer)

   3. Abstract nouns (e.g., accomplishment, satisfaction, affection)

B. Complex sentences that contain major types of subordinate clauses

   1. Adverbial (e.g., *When people exercise*, they lose weight.)

   2. Relative (e.g., People *who exercise* are happier.)

   3. Nominal (e.g., I believe *it's better to relax at home.*)

Before the students begin writing the essays in which they argue their own point of view and attempt to convince others to agree with them, the speech-language pathologist engages the entire group in a series of brainstorming sessions, with each session lasting about 30 minutes. During the first session, a fundamental question is posed: "How should adolescents in the 8th grade spend their afterschool leisure hours?" The two opposing points of view quickly surface. A student representative from each subgroup is asked to come to the white board and make two columns, marked "Reasons For" and "Reasons Against" their point of view. Thus, each subgroup is expected not only to argue in favor of its own point of view, but also to consider the opposite point of view. Next, the representative will ask each member of the subgroup to contribute at least one reason under each column, which then is written on the white board. During this process, another student in the subgroup, the recorder, will be asked to copy the information from the white board into a document to be stored on a laptop computer. The document then will be saved and later modified when the subgroup meets again. During subsequent brainstorming sessions, the students in each subgroup will be expected to add to the list of items under the two columns and to do so by collecting facts from authoritative sources. For example, one subgroup may locate scientific evidence that indicates how physical activity can increase the body's strength and flexibility, build endurance, control weight, maintain blood pressure, and improve sleep. In contrast, the subgroup favoring more sedentary activities may locate scientific evidence indicating that laughter that occurs when talking on the phone with friends can increase endorphins in the brain, leading to feelings of well-being and relaxation. This subgroup also reports a study indicating that time spent talking with others can increase one's social network, providing the opportunity to gain emotional support, collaborate on homework assignments, plan recreational outings, and build solidarity with peers. During the process of reading topic-related articles, an additional benefit is that students are likely to encounter literate vocabulary (e.g., *contentment, coordination, encouragement, metabolism*) that they can then incorporate into their lists and later into their persuasive essays.

After each subgroup has completed its list of items both for and against their point of view, they edit their document, making sure that all points are written in full sentences that are grammatically correct and free of spelling errors. This presents an opportunity for the students with SLI to focus on the production of complex sentences containing literate vocabulary. For example, with guidance from the speech-language pathologist, the following three sentences could be combined into the fourth more efficient sentence, which contains an embedded subordinate clause and a technical term (*hypertension*).

1. Walking home from school every day is good exercise.

2. Walking helps you lose weight.

3. Losing weight can prevent hypertension.

4. Walking [GER] home from school every day is [MC] good exercise because it helps [ADV] you lose [INF] weight, which can prevent [ADV] hypertension.

Next, they are asked to share their information with the entire group by having different members of the subgroup take turns reading each point aloud from the printed document. After each group has had its turn, an open discussion will occur in which all students are encouraged to make comments, ask questions, and express their opinions respectfully.

Following these brainstorming and discussion sessions, students will be asked to write their essays, using a graphic organizer that provides an outline of the essential features of a strong persuasive argument. An example of such a tool is shown here.

1. State the topic and explain why it is controversial.

2. State your own opinion clearly.

3. Give at least three different reasons for your opinion.

4. State what other people believe (the other side of the controversy).

5. Try to explain why other people believe that way.

6. Summarize your opinion and conclude the essay.

In addition, students will be reminded to attend to the following points:

1. Use full sentences with correct grammar and spelling.

2. Use words that are precise, accurate, and engaging.

It is expected that students will need time to write, edit, and revise their essays before the final product is ready to be read by their health teacher and classmates. Because good writing requires patience and persistence, students should be encouraged to approach the task systematically and to remember that the goal is to produce an essay that will influence others. It also can be expected that students may change their minds as they work on their essays, tempering their views after they have considered the evidence on both sides of the controversy. This should be encouraged because it means that the students are grappling with the complexities of the topic and are realizing that few issues are as simple and "black or white" as they first may appear. Indeed, when students move from an extreme position to one that is more balanced and flexible, it shows that they have benefited from the experience of debating an issue and attempting to persuade others.

CHAPTER 9

Bringing It All Together: The School Newspaper

From each according to his ability, to each according to his needs.

Karl Marx

The purpose of this chapter is to describe a procedure for implementing language intervention in an integrative fashion that addresses the genres that have been discussed in this book: conversational, narrative, expository, and persuasive. This approach is designed to be carried out in a middle school or high school journalism class where students with diverse linguistic and cognitive strengths and weaknesses are assigned to work together to produce a school newspaper. Working closely with the journalism teacher, the speech-language pathologist serves as an informed scaffold, assisting students with language disorders or weak language skills to succeed in ecologically valid contexts. The procedure calls upon the students to use their spoken and written language skills as they prepare appropriate material to be printed in each main section of the newspaper. An explanation of how to conduct this type of language intervention is offered, accompanied by some hypothetical examples.

WORK GROUP SCENARIO

At the beginning of the school year, 24 students in an 8th-grade journalism class are assigned to six individual work groups or teams of four students each. At least one student in each group has a language disorder or weak language skills, while the others have average or above average language abilities. Each group is assigned to work on a different section of the newspaper for five consecutive weeks. The sections are titled: (1) "Sports, Weather, and Current Events," (2) "People in Our Community," (3) "One Family's Saga: A Novel," (4) "Food, Clothing, and Lifestyle," (5) "Entertainment," and (6) "Letters to the Editor." During each 5-week assignment, students will produce an article, set of articles, or chapter that pertains to their section to be included in an electronic or printed edition of the newspaper that will be published regularly throughout the school year and made available to the entire school. After each assignment has concluded, each student will rotate to a new group and will work on a new section of the newspaper with a new set of classmates. Thus, each student will participate on six different teams throughout the year, having the opportunity to learn about different topics, use different genres, and adjust to the personalities and communication styles of different peers, building spoken and written language skills in relevant social and academic contexts.

Because the newspaper is designed to inform, entertain, and convince the readership, it has the quality of authenticity and can be expected to motivate the students who are responsible for producing it to use their best spoken and written language skills. For example, students will be expected to discuss with their team members what topics to write about, to decide who will perform what tasks, to formulate questions that could be asked during an interview, to transcribe interviews, and to edit each other's work.

In addition, it will be important for the speech-language pathologist to attempt to build on each student's strengths so that all participants will have the opportunity to be recognized as making a unique and valued contribution to the team effort. For example, those with artistic talent or an interest in photography could be asked to illustrate the various sections, drawing pictures or taking digital photos of, for example, athletes (e.g., the captain of the cross-country team), weather conditions (e.g., a rain storm that flooded the school's basement), foods (e.g., cakes that were prepared by students for a charity bake sale), or classmates (e.g., the winners of a dance contest). Moreover, those who enjoy comics could illustrate humorous (but kind) anecdotes told by peers, to be included in the entertainment section.

Although the speech-language pathologist, working closely with the journalism teacher, continuously provides structure, support, and guidance —particularly for adolescents with language disorders—the students are expected to assume increasing amounts of responsibility and independence as they move through the school year, eventually having the opportunity to work with six different groups. For example, as their language and social skills improve, they will be asked to edit each other's work, a task that requires attention to detail, tactfulness, a positive attitude, and the ability to read and write proficiently. Editing also offers the opportunity to develop students' metalinguistic competence and their skill at critically evaluating the content and style of an article. To ensure a successful editing experience for both the editor and the author, students could be provided with a written outline or graphic organizer that lists certain features to address, beginning with positive comments (e.g., "Here's what I like about your story") before offering constructive feedback (e.g., "Here's what I think you might change"), with each of these headings followed by two or three numbered lines for the editor's comments to be inserted.

SECTIONS OF THE NEWSPAPER

The six sections of the hypothetical school newspaper are described here, along with an explanation of the goals, genres, and activities that are associated with each.

1. Sports, Weather, and Current Events

This section would involve the factual reporting of recent events affecting the school such as the outcome of a cross-country meet, a rain storm that flooded the school's basement, or students' efforts to collect canned foods for impoverished people living in the community. The goal would be to develop students' ability to report the details of such events in an accurate, clear, and organized fashion. Given the factual nature of this section, the articles would be written primarily in the expository genre. However, conversational and persuasive discourse also would be called upon as students discuss and decide among themselves which events to cover, who to interview about those events, and what questions to ask. Additionally, their ability to speak with clarity, precision, and efficiency will be called upon as they interview people such as the cross-country coach, custodian, or secretary, asking questions to elicit detailed explanations. For example, if interviewing the coach, a student might proceed as follows:

1. "I understand that the team finished 8th at the state meet. Did you expect this would happen? Why or why not?"

2. "How do you think the athletes felt about their performance this year?"

3. "What do you think they could do differently next year?"

Similarly, the custodian might be questioned in the following manner:

1. "How much water actually got into the basement?"

2. "How did it get in there? Did someone leave the window open?"

3. "How will the school get the water out of the basement?"

If interviewing the secretary, the following questions might be asked:

1. "Could you tell me how many cans of food the 6th-grade class has collected?"

2. "And how many cans have the 7th- and 8th-grade classes collected?"

3. "Which class do you think will collect the most cans by next week?"

Before adolescents with language disorders are assigned to interview the adults, it will be necessary for them to work closely with the speech-language pathologist and their peers as they prepare their list of statements and questions, typing them into a word processing program on a laptop computer, modifying them for appropriateness, and printing out the final version to be used during the actual interview. These activities are beneficial because they provide an opportunity for students to use complex syntax and literate vocabulary as they speak to authority figures during the interviews. For example, they might ask questions such as, "In your opinion, which team is most likely to win the regional meet?" and "Why do you think they will win?"

It will be important also to ensure that students are comfortable using a microphone and audio recorder and know how to transcribe the interview accurately and completely so that their report reflects what the adult speaker actually said. An adolescent with a language disorder could be paired up with a peer with typical language development when conducting the interview and transcribing the audio recording.

2. People in Our Community

For this section, students could interview a wide range of people who have interesting stories to tell. Examples might include a retired teacher who began working at the school 40 years ago, a fireman who rescued a family from a burning apartment, or a musician who plays Czech folk tunes using different types of flutes and mandolins. The goals would be to develop students' ability to elicit engaging stories from people in a manner that is respectful and sensitive to differences in age, experience, and knowledge, and to encourage students to use complex syntax and literate vocabulary during the interviews. As they transcribe their interviews, students would be expected to write down exactly what a speaker has said, striving for accuracy and objectivity, an opportunity for them to learn about the importance of truth in journalism.

A variety of genres would be called upon, including conversational, expository, and persuasive as the students discuss and decide among themselves how to interview each individual and what questions to ask, and to report the outcome of their efforts. Additionally, it is likely that the interviews will elicit narratives, as for example, when the retired teacher tells a story about a day when her students surprised her by dressing up like the characters from the Shakespearean play they were studying in English class. In transcribing the interviews, students may learn about the subtle features of a good story, including such things as the teacher's use of humor, visual imagery, and sound effects.

3. One Family's Saga: A Novel

This section of the newspaper would provide students an opportunity to work together on a creative writing project, in which narrative discourse would be the predominant genre. At the beginning of the school year, the assigned work group would create a fictional family of adults, children, and pets. For example, the family, "the Arnolds," might consist of a divorced mother who is a yoga instructor; her elderly father who is a retired police officer; two teenage daughters, Chloe (age 18) and Claire (age 16); twin sons, Rusty and Roy (age 10); and three dogs, Rocky, Fiona, and Clover, who were adopted from the Humane Society. During the school year, each work group would write a new chapter about the family and the joys and challenges they experience as they go through life. Each chapter might focus on different characters. For example, chapters might center on the mother taking up a new hobby, ballroom dancing; the grandfather attending his 50th high school reunion, reconnecting with an old girlfriend; Chloe working part time as a waitress; Claire learning to drive; Rusty and Roy spending the summer in Ohio with their father; and the dogs escaping from the backyard, setting off a frantic neighborhood search and mysteriously returning one week later.

The goal of this activity would be for students to write narratives that are original and entertaining by including elements of humor, irony, realism, sarcasm, surprise, elation, disappointment, suspense, and problem solving, paying special attention to the thoughts and feelings of the characters. Students who are especially creative could be encouraged to make up plots, subplots, and the lines that the characters might speak, while those who are attentive listeners and good spellers could type the story into the computer program, where it could be saved and modified as the group makes progress during their five-week assignment. Students who enjoy drawing pictures could illustrate the characters and the situations in which they find themselves. Other students may serve as editors who carefully review each chapter before it is published, tactfully making suggestions to the author to improve the story and its readability. Throughout these activities, adolescents with language disorders must be closely supported, for example, as they suggest the lines that a character might utter. For example, "At home, Chloe often made sarcastic comments to her sister, such as, 'That was the biggest tip (25 cents) I ever got!!'"

To maintain students' motivation, each edition of the newspaper would contain a new chapter about the family. Then, at the end of the school year, all of the chapters could be compiled into a novel that is printed, illustrated, and bound, with multiple copies produced and made available for purchase or for check out at the school library.

4. Food, Clothing, and Lifestyle

This section of the newspaper could include information about favorite foods, popular clothing styles, preferred leisure activities, and other items of interest that are suggested by the students themselves. Possible topics might include how to make certain desserts, how to dress for a football game versus a school dance, the best places in town to go skate boarding, or the use of slang expressions by people of different ages.

The goal would be for students to provide accurate information, written in a clear and engaging manner, primarily in the expository genre. For example, a student with a language disorder who enjoys desserts could be asked to submit a recipe for his favorite cake, written in his own words. Jake, a 14-year-old boy, decides to submit a recipe for Poke 'n Pour Ginger Cake, which he describes as "Awesome!" After listing the ingredients and their required amounts (2¼ cups of flour, ¾ cup of brown sugar, 2 teaspoons of cinnamon, 1 teaspoon of ginger, etc.), Jake would need to explain the steps of setting the oven to the proper temperature, preparing the cake pan, mixing the ingredients, and pouring the batter into the pan. Next, he would need to explain how long to bake the cake and how to determine when it is ready to come out of the oven. Finally, he would need to describe how to make the hot butter sauce and how and when to pour it over the cake after it comes out of the oven. Although Jake is encouraged to refer to a recipe in a cookbook, the manner in which he explains the procedures for making the cake must come from his own knowledge base, to avoid plagiarism. For the cake to be a success when others try his recipe, he must include all ingredients and explain all steps accurately. Additionally, it may be useful to engage Jake in some perspective taking activities to promote awareness of the effectiveness of his communication. For example, to encourage this awareness, the speech-language pathologist might say to Jake, "You said to add the salt. But I don't know how much to add. What if I put in too much?"

Alternatively, a student with a language disorder who is interested in learning about slang expressions might interview people of different ages, such as a high school principal, football coach, librarian, or other students at the school who represent various cliques. This activity could provide an opportunity for the student to work with a peer as they contact potential interviewees, formulate their questions, conduct the interviews, operate the audio recording equipment, transcribe the interviews, and write up their report. They also may gain insight into fascinating aspects of language such as the origins of slang terms, the reasons why people use them, and how their use changes over time. Upon interviewing the principal, for example, a former surfer who grew up in Southern California, they may learn about terms such as beach bunny, hang ten, Neptune cocktail, selling Buicks, shoot the curl, gnarly tube ride, and wipe-out. After interviewing the principal, they may be motivated to interview other adults, such as another student's father, a long-distance truck driver, who provides a detailed explanation of the meaning and use of terms such as bears, donuts, dusting, lollipop, and slappers.

5. Entertainment

This section could include reviews of movies, plays, concerts, or other creative events the students enjoy, including those performed by their classmates such as the school's production of *The Miracle Worker*, a Valentine's Day concert sung by the Glee Club, or the marching band's half-time show at a recent football game. Emphasizing expository discourse, it offers an opportunity for students to evaluate and write about the efforts of others, noting as many positives as possible and couching their criticisms in the kindest of terms, always striving for fairness, compassion, and constructiveness.

An advice column could also be included in this section where, for example, students submit short articles, based on library research or their own experience, that focus on topics such as tips for babysitting young children, how to prevent kitchen fires, rules of the road for riding a bicycle on city streets, or the "Five Most Important Things to Know" about any number of topics (e.g., house-sitting while a neighbor is on vacation, operating a gas-powered lawn mower, preparing a holiday dinner, reporting a stolen bicycle, or backpacking in the wilderness).

Students with language disorders who are working to build their own use of complex syntax at the sentential level might be encouraged to make up a quiz that covers the content that other students have written in their essays. For example, working with the speech-language pathologist, two adolescents with SLI might construct the following questions, both of which are complex sentences containing adverbial clauses and literate vocabulary:

1. When a person goes backpacking, what is one essential survival tool?
   a. Compass
   b. Comic book
   c. Swim suit
   d. Book of stamps

2. Before a family departs for a backpacking trip, what should they do?
   a. Clean out the refrigerator and turn it off.
   b. Tell their friends exactly where they are going.
   c. Renew their subscription to *Field and Stream* magazine.
   d. Take their clothes to the laundromat to be dry cleaned.

Readers of the article then could test their understanding by answering the questions and checking their answers on the next page of the newspaper.

6. Letters to the Editor

This section of the newspaper would emphasize the persuasive genre. Goals would address students' ability to use complex syntax and literate vocabulary, while attempting to convince other people to accept certain beliefs or to perform specific actions. Students who are assigned to this section could ask their classmates to submit letters on a controversial topic that is of interest to others at their school. Topics might include, for example, if students should be allowed to use cell phones in class, if students should be required to wear school uniforms, or if teachers should contact parents when students perform poorly on exams or projects. When requesting submissions, the student editors could explain that only the strongest letters will be published, and that in deciding which letters to accept, they will be using the following checklist to evaluate each one:

1. States the topic and explains why it is controversial.

2. States the author's own opinion clearly.

3. Gives at least three different reasons for the author's opinion.

4. States what other people believe (the other side of the controversy).

5. Tries to explain why other people believe that way.

6. Summarizes the author's opinion and concludes the letter.

7. Uses full sentences with correct grammar and spelling.

8. Uses words that are precise, accurate, and engaging.

This activity places the editors in the position of critically evaluating their peers' persuasive writing, necessitating that they read the letters carefully, understand the content, and examine them for the essential elements, using the checklist to assist them in this process. This could be a worthwhile learning activity, especially when students have the opportunity to review strong letters. By encouraging them to pay attention to the critical elements of a persuasive letter, students may improve their own writing skills.

As an example, the editors might evaluate the following letter, written by an 8th-grade girl, Willow, and her classmates and published in a local newspaper ("Teachers Need to Be Healthy," 2009). The letter concerns a ban on the consumption of junk food at a school, and the controversy centers on whether or not the ban, directed at students, should also include teachers. Willow and her classmates wrote as follows:

> We think that the ban of junk foods in schools should include teachers. Sodas and other junk foods are just as unhealthy for teachers as they are for students. The teachers need to set a good example for the students. If students see that the ban on junk food includes teachers as well as themselves, they might be more willing to go along with the ban. To have a mind and body that functions the best they can, you need to eat the proper amount of nutrients. You do not get these nutrients from junk foods and soda. Because of this, you do not function as well as you could. We think it is important for teachers to have healthy bodies and minds, so that they will teach the students better than otherwise. If teachers eat or drink junk food or soda, they will not teach as well. If the teachers really cannot live without the junk food, they can very easily just eat it at their homes. It should not be that hard for them to wait the seven or eight hours that their jobs take up to eat junk food if they need it that badly. After all, students can.

In reviewing a persuasive letter such as this, students with language disorders may benefit by focusing their attention on the last two points (#7 and #8), determining whether sentences are well constructed and whether appropriate words are used. With the speech-language pathologist acting as a scaffold, they could be encouraged to rewrite any sentences that are incomplete or contain grammatical errors or misspelled words and to substitute more appropriate words, with the goal of assisting the author to improve the letter. They also could be encouraged to identify sentences that contain different types of subordinate clauses and to discuss with the speech-language pathologist how those clauses improve the sentence by adding specific pieces of information. For example, the following sentence from Willow's letter contains three subordinate clauses, one of which [NOM] is embedded into another [ADV]:

> If students see [ADV] that the ban on junk food includes [NOM] teachers as well as themselves, they might be more willing [MC] to go [INF] along with the ban.

After discussing how the adverbial clause in this sentence communicates a certain condition, they might discuss how the metacognitive verb *see* introduces the nominal clause and how both of those subordinate clauses support and modify the main clause. By examining the main clause in isolation (i.e., "they might be more willing to go along with the ban") and comparing it with the full sentence, students might be assisted to understand the role of subordinate clauses in providing essential information in a clear, precise, and efficient manner.

CONCLUSIONS

This chapter has offered suggestions for ways to motivate students to use strong spoken and written language skills for the purpose of publishing a school newspaper. Given the growing popularity of online publishing (along with shrinking school budgets for paper supplies), students may enjoy distributing electronic copies of the newspaper to their classmates, teachers, family members, and friends.

Collaboration between the speech-language pathologist and the journalism teacher and between adolescents with varying strengths and weaknesses in language and cognition has been emphasized. In working together for a genuine purpose, adolescents may rise to the occasion by tapping into their own competencies and employing complex syntax, literate vocabulary, and appropriate pragmatic skills in relevant social and academic contexts.

PART II

Grammar Review and Exercises

CHAPTER 10

Types of Words and Phrases

*T*raditional parts of speech, or "word classes," are nouns, pronouns, adjectives, verbs, adverbs, prepositions, particles, conjunctions, articles, and interjections (Crews, 1977; Quirk & Greenbaum, 1973). This is an ancient but useful method of classifying words that was introduced by the Greek philosopher Aristotle (384–322 BC). Aristotle sought to understand how different words function to express different meanings (*Grammar: Parts of speech [2009]* http://eslus.com/LESSONS/GRAMMAR/POS/pos1.htm).

PARTS OF SPEECH

Nouns

A noun is often described as a "person, place, or thing" (e.g., *dog, cat, house, tree, car*). Nouns can be pluralized (e.g., *dogs, cats, houses, trees, cars*). They also can be preceded by an article (e.g., *a, an, the, some*). A proper noun is the name of a specific person, place, or thing (e.g., John Smith, Chicago, Tugman Park, etc.).

Pronouns

A pronoun represents a noun. There are many types of pronouns, such as personal, possessive, demonstrative, reflexive, relative, indefinite, and interrogative.

1. Personal pronoun: Refers to people or animals and can substitute for specific names of those things (e.g., *I, you, me, he, she, we, they*)

2. Possessive pronoun: Used in place of a noun and implies ownership (e.g., *his* house, *her* mother, *their* books).

3. Demonstrative pronoun: Refers to people, animals, or objects and singles out what they refer to (e.g., *this, these, those, that*; *this* baby is cute; *that* cat is Puff; *those* are Mary's books; *these* shoes are mine).

4. Reflexive pronoun: Refers back to the subject of the sentence (e.g., *himself, herself, themselves, itself, ourselves, yourself*). For example, Mary helped *herself*; Jim and Joe taught *themselves*.

5. Relative pronoun: Introduces a relative clause, which tells about a subject or an object. For example, the boy *who* is late is my brother; the donut *that* you ate was chocolate; you bought the cake *that* was orange; my sister is the one *who* is happy.

6. Indefinite pronoun: Does not specify a specific person, animal, or thing, but refers to something more general (e.g., *anybody, anyone, one, each, any, everything, everyone, some, all, something, somebody, someone*). Other indefinite pronouns include *what, which, who*, and *whose* (when they are not introducing a relative clause). For example, she knows *what* to do; I know *who* will win; I know *which* cat is mine.

7. Interrogative pronoun: Initiates a question (e.g., *who, what, why, when, how, whom, whose, which*). For example, *What* time is it? *How* are you? *Whose* dog is this?

Adjectives

An adjective describes or modifies a noun (e.g., *old, red, big, happy*). Adjectives can be made comparative and superlative (e.g., the *bigger* cake, the *highest* mountain). Other types of words cannot be made comparative or superlative.

Verbs

A verb expresses action (e.g., *run, jump, fall*) or state of being (e.g., *think, feel, know, believe*). Verbs tell you about the subject of the sentence and can express **simple** present, past, or future tense, as in the following examples, where "John" is the subject:

John runs three miles every day. (simple present tense)

John ran three miles yesterday. (simple past tense)

John will run three miles tomorrow. (simple future tense)

In addition to the simple present, past, or future tense of the verb, as in the examples above, there is the **progressive** form of the verb, as in the following examples where Bob is the subject:

> Bob is driving the van today. (present progressive tense)

> Bob was driving the van yesterday. (past progressive tense)

> Bob will be driving the van tomorrow. (future progressive tense)

Finally, in addition to the simple and progressive verb forms, there is the **perfect** form which involves the notion of verb **aspect**. Aspect indicates "the point of time from which an action is seen to take place" (Jarvie, 2007, p. 37). This can involve the present, past, or future aspect, as in the following examples, where Tom is the subject:

> Tom has lived in Chicago for 20 years. (present perfect tense)

> Tom had lived in Chicago for 20 years. (past perfect tense)

> Tom will have lived in Chicago for 20 years next Christmas. (future perfect tense)

Verb Types

There are many types of verbs.

1. Main verb: A sentence must have a main verb. The main verb is most directly related to the subject of the sentence (e.g., Jill *wants* an apple; Bob *runs* fast). Main verbs can express different tenses—past, present, and future. Two types of past tense verbs are past regular and past irregular. Past regular verbs add -ed (e.g., yesterday, the boy *walked*; the boy *talked*; the boy *jumped*). Past irregular verbs take an unpredictable form and do not add -ed (e.g., *ran, wrote, drove, fell, ate*).

2. Copula verb: This is the verb *to be* in its various forms (*is, are, am, was, were, will be*). For example, the ball *is* red; Bill *was* a cowboy; they *are* spooky; we *were* children. The copula is a finite verb that links or joins the subject of the sentence to the predicate. It is the main verb of the clause. It is marked for person (1st, 2nd, 3rd), tense (present, past, future), and number (singular, plural; Table 10–1)

3. Auxiliary verb: These are helping verbs that combine with other verbs and work with the main verb (e.g., he *is* swimming; they *are* running; we *had been* eating). The auxiliary verb (*is, are*) expresses person (first, second, third), tense (past, present, future), and number (singular, plural). For example, he *was* swimming; they *were* running. Other auxiliary verbs include *can, will,* and *do*. For example, I *can* read this; she *will* be late; *don't* forget to vote (see Table 10–1.)

TABLE 10–1. How Copula and Auxiliary Verbs Are Marked for Person (1st, 2nd, 3rd), Tense (Past, Present, Future), and Number (Singular, Plural)

| Number | Person | TENSE | | |
		Present	Past	Future
		Copula Verb		
Singular	**1st**	I am happy.	I was happy.	I will be happy.
	2nd	You are happy.	You were happy.	You will be happy.
	3rd	She/he is happy.	She/he was happy	She/he will be happy.
Plural	**1st**	We are happy.	We were happy.	We will be happy.
	2nd	You are happy.	You were happy.	You will be happy.
	3rd	They are happy.	They were happy.	They will be happy.
		Auxiliary Verb		
Singular	**1st**	I am going.	I was going.	I will be going.
	2nd	You are going.	You were going.	You will be going.
	3rd	She/he is going.	She/he was going.	She/he will be going.
Plural	**1st**	We are going.	We were going.	We will be going.
	2nd	You are going.	You were going.	You will be going.
	3rd	They are going.	They were going.	They will be going.

4. Modal verb: This is a special type of auxiliary verb. Modal verbs help to express the mood or attitude of the speaker, or special conditions (e.g., *might, could, should, may, need, will, ought to, used to, would, shall, must*). For example, you *might* like the new book; he *should* do his work; we *may* go shopping tomorrow. Modals can express a mood of uncertainty (e.g., you *might* like the movie) or of certainty (e.g., you *must* see the movie).

5. Finite verb: A verb that is marked for person (1st, 2nd, 3rd), tense (past, present, future), and number (singular, plural):

   She *walked* to the store yesterday.

   He *will walk* to the store tomorrow.

   They *are walking* to the store right now.

   He/she/it *walks*; I walk; they *walk* every day.

   Mary *has walked* 16 miles today.

6. Nonfinite verb: A verb that is unmarked for person, tense, and number. They include infinitives, gerunds, and participles.

   A. Infinitive: This is a verb in its unmarked form, as one would find it in the dictionary. It is often preceded by "to" (e.g., *to go, to run, to dance, to play*). For example, I wanted *to go* home; the teenagers planned *to dance* all night. Sometimes *to* is omitted (e.g., I saw the lion *eat* the meat).

   B. Gerund: This verb ends with -ing and acts like a noun (e.g., *swimming* is good exercise; *smoking* is bad for you; they enjoy *knitting*; her hobbies are *fishing* and *embroidering*).

   C. Participle: This verb ends in -ing, -ed, or -en, and acts like an adjective (e.g., the *swimming* boy got to shore; the *crooked* fence fell down; the *broken* cup was thrown out.)

Adverbs

An adverb modifies or describes a verb (e.g., he drove *slowly;* the rain fell *quietly*; she ran *quickly*). Adverbs often end in the suffix -ly (e.g., *nicely, quickly, hastily, slowly*) but not always (e.g., I will work *now*). There are many types of adverbs, for example:

1. Adverb of time: This answers the question "when." For example, when did she run? She ran *early*. Other examples include *later, tonight, yesterday, before, after, now*.

2. Adverb of place: This answers the question "where." For example, where did she run? She ran *everywhere*. Other examples include *anywhere, here, somewhere, there*.

3. Adverb of manner: This answers the question "how?" For example, how did she drive? She drove *cautiously*. Other examples include *carefully, jokingly, kindly, slowly*.

4. Adverb of magnitude: This expresses the degree of size, amount, or intensity (e.g., *slightly, somewhat, rather, quite, decidedly, extremely, unusually*).

5. Adverb of likelihood: This expresses the degree of probability (e.g., *absolutely, certainly, definitely, maybe, perhaps, positively, possibly, probably*).

Adverbs can modify other types of words besides verbs. For example, they can modify adjectives (e.g., the *very* pretty coat) and other adverbs (e.g., *early* yesterday morning; she ran *very* quickly). In fact, any modifier that is not an adjective or an article is probably an adverb.

Prepositions

A preposition is a small word such as to, in, under, over, into, on, above. These words introduce a prepositional phrase (e.g., I went *to the store*; I put it *on the shelf*; the ball rolled *under the bed*). A prepositional phrase consists of a preposition and its object.

Particles

A particle looks like a preposition but does not act like one. Particles are small words such as up, down, off, in, out that co-occur with specific verbs as in look up, roll down, turn off, let in, throw out, cut up, wear out. Particles, unlike prepositions, can sometimes shift their position to the right of the object. For example, he looked *up* the number/he looked the number *up*; she rolled *down* the window/she rolled the window *down*; he turned *off* the TV/he turned the TV *off*; she let *in* the cat/she let the cat *in*; he threw *out* the trash/he threw the trash *out*.

Conjunctions

A conjunction is a small word that connects other words (within a clause) or connects clauses (within a sentence). They are also called *connectives* (e.g., and, but, or, for, so, yet, although). For example, he likes ham *and* eggs; I'll take blue *or* red; he doesn't like jam *but* she does. There are three major types of conjunctions: coordinate, subordinate, and correlative.

1. Coordinate (e.g., and, but, for, or, so, yet). These conjunctions introduce an independent (main) clause (e.g., I like strawberry *but* Bill likes chocolate). Examples include and, but, for, or, so, and yet. Coordinate conjunctions often signal a main clause, one that could stand by itself and make sense (e.g., I went shopping, *and* Mary stayed home).

2. Subordinate (e.g., after, although, unless). These conjunctions introduce a dependent (subordinate) clause (e.g., *although* it was raining, we went for a walk). Subordinate conjunctions signal a dependent (subordinate) clause, a clause that usually cannot stand alone and make sense (e.g., *after* the rain stopped, we went outside). Other examples of subordinate conjunctions include the following: as, as if, as long as, as soon as, as though, because, before, how, if, in order that, provided that, since, that, though, till, until, when, whenever, where, wherever, while, so that. Some of these conjunctions also may introduce a phrase rather than a clause (e.g., *Because of his teacher's encouragement*, he applied for a scholarship).

3. Correlative (e.g., both . . . and; either . . . or; neither . . . nor; not only . . . but also). Correlative conjunctions occur as groups of words within the same clause. For example, I want *both* coffee *and* pie; George wants *not only* chocolate *but also* vanilla; I'll take *either* pizza *or* spaghetti; he likes *neither* pie *nor* cake.

Adverbial Conjuncts

This is a special type of conjunction that introduces a main clause. For example, meanwhile, hence, consequently, accordingly, similarly, conversely, contrastively. These words are frequently found in literate contexts and serve to link ideas in a logical manner. For example, Tim likes Bach; *consequently*, he bought a ticket to the concert.

Articles

An article is a small word that immediately precedes a noun or adjective. The article identifies (or points out) the noun; it doesn't describe it (e.g., *a*, *the*, *an*). For example, *the* dog was old; I want *a* big cookie. Articles are either definite (*the*) or indefinite (*a*, *an*). A definite article identifies a particular object (e.g., *the* dog, *the* girl). An indefinite article doesn't specify any particular object (e.g., I'll take *an* orange; I'd like *a* book).

Interjections

This is an informal expression of emotion (e.g., Ah! Ahah! Good grief! Gosh! Hey! Hurrah! Oh! OK! Ouch! Right! Shh! Ugh! Whew!).

PHRASES

A *phrase* is a small group of words that functions as if it were a specific part of speech (e.g., noun, verb, preposition, etc.). A phrase is a larger unit than a word but a smaller unit than a clause because it lacks a subject-predicate relationship (Crews, 1977; Dumond, 1993; Jarvie, 2007).

The main types of phrases are defined below, followed by examples:

Noun Phrase

Definition: A group of words that contains a noun; it may also contain an article (e.g., *a*, *an*, *the*) and possibly some modifiers.

Examples:

The snowy mountain range (noun = *range*)

A glorious golden field (noun = *field*)

An acrobatic ski jump (noun = *jump*)

Age zero main sequence (noun = *sequence*)

Verb Phrase

Definition: A group of words that contains a verb and possibly some auxiliaries such as modal verbs (e.g., could, should, must).

Examples:

Had been sleeping (main verb = *sleeping*)

Could have been watching (main verb = *watching*)

May have written (main verb = *written*)

Was building (main verb = *building*)

Prepositional Phrase

Definition: A group of words that contains a preposition followed by a noun phrase.

Examples:

Under the rock (preposition = *under*)

Along the winding river (preposition = *along*)

In a colorful clown suit (preposition = *in*)

Over the slippery slope (preposition = *over*)

Prepositional phrases can also post-modify noun phrases:

The sports car *with the silver hub caps* (preposition = *with*)

The very old house *beyond the apple tree* (preposition = *beyond*)

Adjective Phrase

Definition: A group of words that contains an adjective and modifies a noun or noun phrase. The adjective phrase can come either before or after the noun phrase.

Examples:

A *complex and scary* poem (adjectives = *complex, scary*)

An *honest and forthright* mechanic (adjectives = *honest, forthright*)

The dog was *extremely well-behaved* (adjective = *well-behaved*)

The house was *old and dilapidated* (adjectives = *old, dilapidated*)

Adverb Phrase

Definition A: A group of words that contains an adverb that modifies another adverb; as a unit, those words work together to modify a verb in the sentence.

Examples:

She ran *rather quickly* down the street (the adverb *rather* modifies the adverb *quickly*; as a unit, the adverb phrase modifies the verb *ran*)

She counted the money *quite carefully* (the adverb *quite* modifies the adverb *carefully*; as a unit, the adverb phrase modifies the verb *counted*)

He greeted the diners *most cheerfully* (the adverb *most* modifies the adverb *cheerfully*; as a unit, the adverb phrase modifies the verb *greeted*)

He opened the door *somewhat cautiously* (the adverb *somewhat* modifies the adverb *cautiously*; as a unit, the adverb phrase modifies the verb *opened*)

Definition B: An adverb phrase can also begin with a subordinate conjunction and modify a verb. Unlike an adverbial clause (see Chapter 11), an adverb phrase does not contain a verb.

Examples:

He ordered coffee *after midnight* (the adverb phrase tells **when** he ordered coffee)

She will sleep *until the dawn* (the adverb phrase tells **how long** she will sleep)

Because of the rain, they stayed home (the adverb phrase tells **why** they stayed home)

He ate lunch *before noon* (the adverb phrase tells **when** he ate)

They have lived in California *since the earthquake of 1971.*

EXERCISES: IDENTIFYING TYPES OF WORDS

Exercise 10–1. Identifying Words in Passages

In passages 1–6, circle all of the nouns including *gerunds* and *proper nouns* (but not pronouns).

1. Computers can do lots of things. They can add millions of numbers in the twinkling of an eye. They can outwit chess grandmasters. They can guide weapons to their targets. They can book you onto a plane between a guitar-strumming nun and a nonsmoking physics professor. Some can even play the bongos. That's quite a variety! So if we're going to talk about computers, we'd better decide right now which of them we're going to look at, and how (Feynman, 1996, p. 1).

2. Most of the luxuries, and many of the so-called comforts of life, are not only not indispensable, but positive hindrances to the elevation of mankind. With respect to luxuries and comforts, the wisest have ever lived a more simple and meager life than the poor. The ancient philosophers, Chinese, Hindoo, Persian, and Greek, were a class than which none has been poorer in outward riches, none so rich in inward (Thoreau, 2004, p. 14).

3. For a French parent, education is everything. The child must have as many and as important certificates of academic attainment as possible. In American and British business life, experience counts. In French life, the right education and the right certificates count. This is why some experienced American and British teachers wishing to work in France are horrified to find their experience downgraded because they do not have the equivalent degree certificate to the French one (Tomalin, 2003, p. 93).

4. There are two kinds of knowledge. One is the everyday kind of knowledge we have of the world, which we get through our senses (usually called "empirical" knowledge). Plato thought that this kind

of knowledge was useful enough for ordinary people to go about their everyday lives. But it wasn't the real thing. Like Heraclitus, Pythagoras, and maybe Socrates, Plato thought that the empirical world was a kind of illusion, a veil that hid the real truth from us (Robinson & Groves, 2005, p. 62).

5. Plato was probably the greatest philosopher of all time, and the first to collect all sorts of different ideas and arguments into books that everyone can read. He wanted to know about everything and constantly pestered his fellow philosophers for answers to his disturbing questions. He also had resolute ideas of his own, some of which seem sensible enough, and some of which now seem extremely odd. But, from the start, he knew that "doing philosophy" was a very special activity (Robinson & Groves, 2005, p. 3).

6. I propose that educationalists should no longer conceive of children as passive, empty jam jars who need to be stuffed with information, but as independently minded problem solvers who need to be continually challenged. (John Dewey; Robinson & Groves, 2004, p. 111)

In passages 7–12, circle all of the *adjectives* including the *participles*:

7. The legacy of Scotland's tumultuous and often violent history can be found in its extraordinary array of prehistoric sites, religious ruins, and other historic attractions. Today these relics offer visitors intriguing insights into some of the defining battles, heroes, and forgotten worlds of the country's rich and turbulent past (Wilson & Murphy, 2008, p. 274).

8. Once Oregon was thought to be immune to earthquakes. Today we know that we have them in three different flavors—devastating subduction earthquakes like the 1700 catastrophe, deep intraplate earthquakes like the Puget Sound temblors of 1949 and 2001, and sharp local jolts like the Spring Break Quake of 1993 (Sullivan, 2008, p. 67).

9. Some artists are finite draftsmen with meticulous drawing skills. Other artists are storytellers. A few invent a new lens of perception. But Sarkis Antikajian is a painter. His work is a bodacious celebration of brush dipped in paint and spread across canvas. While some painters claim they paint light, Sarkis Antikajian paints energy. He leaves his viewer breathless by the onslaught on his transcription. His masterful use of intense chroma ravishes the visual cortex in a heady embrace. Sarkis wields color with the same bravado employed by the trumpeter Maynard Ferguson when he plays C above high C (Moffet, 2006, pp. 18–19).

10. The ancient Greeks made extensive use of honey in salves and potions, in prepared dishes, to make perfume, as libations for the dead, and to appease the gods. Bee-keepers numbered among their ranks the philosopher Aristotle; for Hippocrates, the father of medicine, honey was a favorite remedy. The followers of Pythagoras lived on a diet of bread and honey—and seemed to far outlive any of their contemporaries (Style, 1993, p. 14).

11. French culture once dominated Western civilization. From about 1650 to about 1920, the upper classes in several countries preferred French to their own native languages. French was the official language for diplomatic negotiations and much government business. The achievements of French writers, artists, architects, and composers were widely admired and imitated. Since then, other cultures have moved to the forefront. English has overtaken French as the most widely spoken language (Harris, 1989, p. 167).

12. Mister Fox was just about famished and thirsty too, when he stole into a vineyard where the sun-ripened grapes were hanging upon a trellis in a tempting show, but too high for him to reach. He took a run and a jump, snapping at the nearest bunch, but missed. Again and again he jumped, only to miss the luscious prize. At last, worn out with his efforts, he retreated, muttering: "Well, I never really

wanted those grapes anyway. I am sure they are sour, and perhaps wormy in the bargain" ("The Fox and the Grapes," Grosset & Dunlap, 1947, p. 14).

In passages 13–17, circle all of the *finite verbs*:

13. Trieste, set on a gulf with rolling hills as a backdrop, is the most important seaport on the northern Adriatic. Because of its geographic position and its history, the cooking of Trieste is eclectic. *Gnocchetti di fegato*, liver dumplings, are a reminder of Austrian ties. Venezia's influence is apparent in its many risotto, including its own version of *risi e bisi*. It also has its own variation of *brodetto*, the fish stew so popular along the entire Italian coastline. Made with local fish, the sauce contains vinegar, wine, and sometimes tomatoes, and is always served with grilled polenta. There are many rich desserts. Typical are *strucoli*, similar to strudel, which like *preniz*, an Easter specialty, are made with a variety of ingredients (Luciano et al., 1991, p. 87).

14. When first I took up my abode in the woods, that is, began to spend my nights as well as days there, which, by accident, was on Independence Day, or the fourth of July, 1845, my house was not finished for winter, but was merely a defense against the rain, without plastering or chimney, the walls being of rough weather-stained boards, with wide chinks, which made it cool at night (Thoreau, 2004, p. 81).

15. The only house I had been the owner of before, if I except a boat, was a tent, which I used occasionally when making excursions in the summer, and this is still rolled up in my garret; but the boat, after passing from hand to hand, has gone down the stream of time. With this more substantial shelter about me, I had made some progress toward settling in the world (Thoreau, 2004, p. 82).

16. Sonja Kovalevsky (1850–1891), earlier known as Sophia Korvin-Krukovsky, was a gifted mathematician. She was born in Moscow to Russian nobility. She left Russia in 1868 because universities were closed to women. She went to Germany because she wished to study with Karl Weierstrass in Berlin. It was said that her early interest in mathematics was due in part to an odd wallpaper that covered her room in a summer house. Fascinated, she spent hours trying to make sense of it. The paper turned out to be lecture notes on higher mathematics purchased by her father during his student days (Smith, 1995, p. 479).

17. In his famous laboratory school at the University of Chicago, children were (and still are) encouraged to solve problems by inventing hypotheses and testing them. Dewey thought that art should be encouraged because it stimulates imaginative "solutions" to its own unique "problems" (Robinson & Groves, 2004, p. 111).

In passages 18–22, circle all of the *adverbs*.

18. Western Iran extends from the border with Armenia and Azerbaijan in the north to the industrial city of Ahvaz near the Gulf. Culturally, it is the most diverse part of Iran, with Azaris, Armenians, Loris, Bakhtiaris, and Kurds among the distinct ethnic groups you'll encounter. Despite this and a wealth of historical, religious, and cultural sights, stunning mountain scenery, and great trekking possibilities, few travelers see more than Tabriz. Pity them, then take advantage of the unspoilt expanses and go yourself (Ham et al., 2006, p. 199).

19. The Middle East is home to some of the world's most significant cities—Jerusalem, Cairo, Damascus, Baghdad, and Istanbul. The ruins of the once similarly epic cities of history—Petra, Persepolis, Ephesus, Palmyra, Baalbek, Leptis Magna, and the bounty of ancient Egypt—also mark the passage of centuries in a region where the ancient world lives and breathes. The landscapes of the region

are equally spellbinding, from the unrivalled seas of sand dunes and palm-fringed lakes in Libya's Sahara desert to the stunning mountains of the north, and the underwater world of the Red Sea (Ham et al., 2006, p. 4).

20. Mt. Fuji is the highest mountain in Japan, and by far the most splendid, but during July and August (the open season) it is not a dauntingly hard climb. An athlete, it is said, could leave home in Tokyo in the morning, reach the peak, and be home in time for dinner. Most people prefer to take it at a more leisurely pace, spending a night at the top and greeting the morning sun with a cry of "*Banzai!*" (Popham, 1992, p. 159).

21. I left the woods for as good a reason as I went there. Perhaps it seemed to me that I had several more lives to live, and could not spare any more time for that one. It is remarkable how easily and insensibly we fall into a particular route, and make a beaten track for ourselves. I had not lived there a week before my feet wore a path from my door to the pond-side; and though it is five or six years since I trod it, it is still quite distinct. It is true, I fear that others may have fallen into it, and so helped to keep it open (Thoreau, 2004, p. 313).

22. John Dewey (1859–1952) was a systematic pragmatist or "instrumentalist" who believed that being "philosophical" really meant being critically intelligent and maintaining a "scientific" approach to human problems. Pragmatists like Dewey were great enthusiasts for the successes of science and its methods of inquiry. Dewey was convinced that philosophy could also play a key role in a creative American democracy by contributing to all kinds of knowledge in ethics, art, education, and the newly emerging social sciences. Like Pierce, Dewey was a theoretical "fallibilist," but still firmly a believer in the real possibility of practical progress in human affairs. Society can only progress if its members are educated to be intelligent and flexible (Robinson & Groves, 2004, p. 111).

In passage 23, circle all of the *prepositions*:

23. The year 1877 was an important one in the study of the planet Mars. The Red Planet came unusually close to Earth, affording astronomers an especially good view. Of particular note was the discovery, by U.S. Naval Observatory astronomer Asaph Hall, of the two moons circling Mars. But most exciting was the report of the Italian astronomer Giovanni Schiaparelli on his observations of a network of linear markings that he termed *canali*. In Italian, the word usually means "grooves" or "channels," but it can also mean "canals" (Chaisson & McMillan, 2005, p. 140).

In passages 24–25, circle all of the *pronouns*:

24. This country, with its institutions, belongs to the people who inhabit it. Whenever they shall grow weary of the existing government, they can exercise their *constitutional* right of amending it, or their *revolutionary* right to dismember, or overthrow it. I cannot be ignorant of the fact that many worthy and patriotic citizens are desirous of having the constitution amended (Emerson, 2009/1841, *Self-Reliance*, p. 41).

25. All the barnyard knew that the hen was indisposed. So one day, the cat decided to pay her a visit of condolence. Creeping up to her nest, the cat in his most sympathetic voice said, "How are you, my dear friend? I was so sorry to hear of your illness. Isn't there something that I can bring you to cheer you up and to help you feel like yourself again?" "Thank you," said the hen. "Please be good enough to leave me in peace, and I have no fear but I shall soon be well."
    Moral: Uninvited guests are often most welcome when they are gone. ("The Cat and the Hen," Grosset & Dunlap, 1947, p. 133).

In passage 26, circle all of the *articles*:

26. Starting in the 1870s, another upheaval in the arts resulted from the development of a new approach to painting called Impressionism.

Young artists rejected the long-accepted, conventional ways of presenting reality. They too were fascinated by recent discoveries in science and experimented with new techniques for capturing the effects of light. Often they used tiny dabs of complementary colors, relying on the viewer's eyes and mind to bring them together and form the desired effect. The Postimpressionist painters of the late 19th and early 20th centuries worked out new ways of seeing that were highly personal. They scorned the old emphasis on reproducing reality as accurately as possible. Instead, they sought to express their own innermost visions and emotions (Harris, 1989, pp. 173–175).

In passages 27–28, circle all of the *conjunctions*:

27. A woman of many gifts, Margaret Fuller (1810–1850) is most aptly remembered as America's first true feminist. In her brief yet fruitful life, she was variously author, editor, literary and social critic, journalist, poet, and revolutionary. She was also one of the few female members of the prestigious Transcendentalist movement, whose ranks included Ralph Waldo Emerson, Henry David Thoreau, Elizabeth Palmer Peabody, Nathaniel Hawthorne, and many other prominent New England intellectuals of the day. As coeditor of the transcendentalist journal, *The Dial*, Fuller was able to give voice to her groundbreaking social critique on woman's place in society, the genesis of the book that was later to become *Woman in the Nineteenth Century* (Pine, 1999, p. 133).

28. When people started to analyze English grammar in the eighteenth century, it seemed logical to look at the language using the terms and distinctions which had proved so useful in studying Latin. English had no word-endings, it seemed. Therefore, it had no "grammar." But of course there is far more to grammar than word-endings. Some languages (such as Chinese) have none at all. English has less than a dozen types of regular ending (and a few irregular ones; Crystal, 2002, p. 22).

Exercise 10–2. Word Classes

For each word that is in bold, indicate its class—noun, pronoun, verb, adjective, adverb, conjunction, or preposition. Write the word next to the class on the lines following the passage.

Many trees **on** campus are not **native to** the **local** area. Eugene can **support** a greater **variety** of trees than many **places because its** **climate** is **moderate** enough to **easily** accommodate **trees** from colder **and** warmer **areas**. This **led** to the **campus** becoming an **arboretum**. However, planting nonnative trees **displaces** local trees. For **future** tree selections on campus, a **stronger emphasis** on native **species** would **eventually** turn the campus **into a richer learning environment**. One student commented **thoughtfully** that **her favorite** tree was the **Eastern black walnut**, near Gerlinger Hall.

Nouns: (11) _____

_____

_____

_____

Pronouns: (2) _____

Verbs: (3) _____

Adjectives: (10) _____

_____

_____

Adverbs: (3) _____

Conjunctions: (2) _____

Prepositions: (3) _____

Exercise 10–3. Pronouns

1. Circle the **reflexive** pronouns: me   you   us   we   ourselves
   him   her   himself

2. Circle the **demonstrative** pronouns: the   it   that   those   these
   their   this

3. Circle the **interrogative** pronouns: he   on   under   what   her
   who   why   must

4. Circle the **possessive** pronouns: her   that   his   their   any   only
   ourselves

5. Circle the **relative** pronouns: who   his   that   their   which
   them   they

Exercise 10–4. Particles versus Prepositions

Circle the *particles*:

1. She threw down the pen.
2. He ran down the hill.
3. They sat on the bench.
4. He filled up his plate.
5. She ran to the door.
6. He took off the brace.

Circle the *prepositions*:

7. He gave away his books.
8. She sat by the river.
9. They moved to Portland.
10. He ate with a fork.
11. She looked at the sea.
12. He ran from the dog.

Exercise 10–5. Adverbs

1. Circle the adverbs of **manner**:   quietly   happily   somewhere   forever   dreamy

2. Circle the adverbs of **time**:   later   pleasantly   lonely   now   everyone   always

3. Circle the adverbs of **place**:   wherever   whenever   forever   somewhere   anywhere

4. Circle the adverbs of **magnitude**:   gleefully   definitely   unusually   slightly

5. Circle the adverbs of **likelihood**:   possibly   joyously   probably   cleverly

Exercise 10–6. Conjunctions

1. Circle the **subordinate** conjunctions: forever   anyway   unless   while   before

2. Circle the **coordinate** conjunctions: and   until   whenever   why   to   but   off

3. Circle the **adverbial conjuncts**:   consequently   because   while   wherever   thus   moreover

Exercise 10–7. Review: Word Classes

Read the following fable. Then identify each type of word listed below by filling in the blanks. List each word only once.

The Lion and the Mouse (Grosset & Dunlap, 1947, pp. 137–138)

A lion was asleep in his den one day, when a mischievous mouse for no reason at all ran across the outstretched paw and up the royal nose of the king of beasts, awakening him from his nap. The mighty beast clapped his paw upon the now thoroughly frightened little creature and would have made an end of him.

"Please," squealed the mouse, "don't kill me. Forgive me this time, O King, and I shall never forget it. A day may come, who knows, when I may do you a good turn to repay your kindness." The lion, smiling at his little prisoner's fright and amused by the thought that so small a creature ever could be of assistance to the king of beasts, let him go.

Not long afterward the lion, while ranging the forest for his prey, was caught in the net which the hunters had set to catch him. He let out a roar that echoed through the forest. Even the mouse heard it, and recognizing the voice of his former preserver and friend, ran to the spot where he lay tangled in the net of ropes.

"Well, your majesty," said the mouse, "I know you did not believe me once when I said I would return a kindness, but here is my chance." And without further ado he set to work to nibble with his sharp little teeth at the ropes that bound the lion. Soon the lion was able to crawl out of the hunter's snare and be free.

Application: No act of kindness, no matter how small, is ever wasted.

Proverb: One good turn deserves another.

List each type of word (list each word only once):

1. List the *nouns*: _____

   _____

   _____

   _____

   _____

2. List the *adjectives* (but not the participles): _____

   _____

   _____

3. List the *participles*: _____

_____

4. List the *verbs*: _____

_____

_____

_____

_____

5. List the *adverbs*: _____

_____

Exercise 10–8. Phrases

In each sentence below, indicate the type of phrase that is bolded. Use the following codes:

NP = noun phrase

VP = verb phrase

PP = prepositional phrase

AJP = adjective phrase

AVP = adverb phrase

_____ 1. The ball rolled **under the apple tree**.

_____ 2. The ranger told the ghost story **quite enthusiastically** to the teenagers.

_____ 3. The hikers **had not yet arrived** back at camp by nightfall.

_____ 4. The two friends sat down together **very cheerfully** to enjoy their dinner.

_____ 5. **The charming old village** overlooked the river.

_____ 6. Marty missed school **because of a stomach ache**.

_____ 7. They **may have eaten** fish tonight for dinner.

_____ 8. The resort specializes **in outdoor entertainment**.

_____ 9. The lion **had been watching** the sparrows peck at the corn cobs.

_____ 10. **The dry, old bread crumbs** had been left by a group of picnickers.

_____ 11. **Ever since Christmas**, Eva has been happy.

_____ 12. There are **several year-round, modernized, and attractive** inns in town.

_____ 13. **Magnetic and electrical fields** may be present.

_____ 14. The French have a holiday entitlement **of five weeks a year**.

_____ 15. There are **many long, steep, and winding** stretches of trail nearby.

_____ 16. **The well-trained and persistent geologists** discovered large ice crystals.

_____ 17. The actor, tired and sick, struggled **rather mightily** to remember his lines.

_____ 18. The **densely wooded mountain** side was a familiar friend to all.

_____ 19. Two crows **were fighting furiously** in the old corn field.

_____ 20. The poem was written in **flowery Victorian** language.

_____ 21. The children knocked on their new neighbor's door **somewhat shyly**.

_____ 22. The athletes **were running** around the track to warm up before the meet.

_____ 23. **Before the race**, she double-knotted her track shoes.

_____ 24. Jimmy was thrilled with the **brand new, shiny, red** bicycle.

_____ 25. **The rain-soaked graduation picnic** was a memorable event.

Exercise 10–9. Verb Tenses

For each of the sentences below, indicate the **verb tense** from the following choices:

A. Past perfect tense

B. Future progressive tense

C. Simple past tense

D. Present perfect tense

E. Simple future tense

F. Past progressive tense

G. Simple present tense

H. Present progressive tense

I. Future perfect tense

_____   1. Yesterday, the Jones family arrived at Heathrow Airport around 2:00 p.m.

_____   2. The direct flight from San Francisco had taken over 11 hours.

_____   3. By 4:00 p.m., they were checking into their hotel in London.

_____   4. Understandably, by early evening, all were feeling tired and hungry.

_____   5. So they went out to a nearby pub for a delicious dinner of fish and chips.

_____   6. By nine o'clock that evening, the family had settled into their room for the night.

_____   7. It is now six o'clock in the morning, their first full day in the UK.

_____   8. Today, the travelers will be taking the train from England to Wales.

_____   9. They will have reached Llandudno, their final destination, by 11:30 a.m.

_____ 10. Now on the train, their son Liam is playing chess with his sister Jessie.

_____ 11. Jessie will eventually win the match, much to Liam's chagrin.

_____ 12. The children's mother, Martha, has just finished reading a short story.

_____ 13. And their father, Bruce, is ordering coffee from the trolley cart.

_____ 14. By two o'clock this afternoon, the Jones family will be enjoying the beach.

_____ 15. By that time, Liam will have forgotten about his loss to Jessie.

_____ 16. And Jessie will be searching for sea shells and colorful rocks.

_____ 17. Liam has just learned the Welsh name for Wales, "Cymu."

_____ 18. Suddenly, Jessie wants a red tee shirt with "Cymu" on the front.

_____ 19. Dad will buy it for her and one for Liam, too.

_____ 20. Soon the Jones family will be walking back to their B & B after a fun-filled day.

CHAPTER 11

Types of Clauses

A clause is a group of words that expresses a specific meaning. Every clause has a subject and a verb. However, the subject is not always present in the surface structure of the clause as in the case of nonfinite clauses (e.g., *swimming across the lake*, the dog grew weary) or coreferential coordinated main clauses (e.g., Patricia enjoyed basketball *but preferred football*). Major types of clauses are main, coordinate, and subordinate. More information on clauses may be found in Crews (1977) and Quirk and Greenbaum (1973).

MAIN, COORDINATE, AND SUBORDINATE CLAUSES

A *main* clause [MC] has one verb (the "main" verb) and can stand by itself as a complete sentence. For example, people *interact* with their environment; pollution *is* harmful to the atmosphere. The main clause often is called the independent clause or the matrix clause. Sometimes a sentence contains two or more main clauses, linked by a coordinate conjunction (e.g., and, but, so). Those clauses are called *coordinate* clauses:

> The Spaniards brought new animals to Mexico, *and* they introduced new trades.

Peru has many resources, *but* it also has many economic challenges.

John ran out of peanut butter, *so* he went to the store.

Sometimes, when two coordinate clauses contain the same subject, the subject is mentioned in the first clause but is deleted in the next one. This is called *ellipsis*:

John made cookies, (John) cleaned up the kitchen, and (John) took a nap.

Coordinate clauses are on equal footing with each other, such that one clause does not dominate the other. In contrast, a *subordinate* (dependent) clause is of lesser status than the main clause and must be attached to the main clause. There are three primary types of finite subordinate clauses: adverbial, relative, and nominal.

1. *Adverbial* [ADV] clauses perform a variety of functions within a sentence by expressing different meanings such as conditionality, reason (cause), manner, time, contrast, comparison, place, and purpose, as in the following examples:

   Less gasoline is used *when more people ride bicycles.* (conditionality)

   Kittens are domestic only *so far as it suits their own needs.* (conditionality)

   They cancelled the lecture *because the professor was ill.* (reason/cause)

   She performed the solo *exactly as she had practiced it.* (manner)

   We bought tickets *as soon as they were available.* (time)

   Some geographers study traffic flow *while others trace human movement.* (contrast)

   She ran the marathon *as though she were flying.* (comparison)

   A long time ago, the continents were not located *where they are today.* (place)

   The migrant farmers traveled *wherever they could find work.* (place)

   He moved to Boston *so that he could become wealthy.* (purpose)

Adverbial clauses often begin with subordinate conjunctions. Examples of subordinate conjunctions that express different meanings are shown here (adapted from Crystal, 1996, p. 205):

Conditionality: as long as, if, in case, unless, supposing, even though, although

Reason/cause: because, since, for

Manner: joyfully, hurriedly, happily, sadly, apprehensively, reluctantly

Time: after, before, since, until, when, while

Comparison: as if, as though, like

Place: where, wherever

Purpose: in order to, so as to

2. *Nominal* [NOM] clauses, often called "complements," complete a thought or express an attitude, belief, or feeling that is introduced by the main clause. They often follow a metacognitive (e.g., know, believe, think) or metalinguistic (e.g., say, tell, ask) verb that occurs in the main clause, as in the following examples:

I'm not sure *who is coming to dinner.*

James told Susan *that he would be home late.*

Some people believe *they need supplements every day.*

Nominal clauses are enclosed in quotation marks when a speaker or writer is reporting exactly what someone has said:

The young boy asked, "*Why should I become a scholar?*"

The judge told Manuel, "*Put away your money.*"

The pronouns that, how, where, whether, whoever, and what often introduce nominal clauses:

She believes *that he is innocent.*

I don't know *how we will manage.*

A teenager's self-image influences *how others see him or her.*

Adolescents are interested in *how their peers perceive them.*

She could not remember *how the candlesticks got broken.*

Please tell me *whether you would like pie or cake for dessert.*

Mom has asked me *what the answer is to the math question.*

3. *Relative* [REL] clauses add precision by describing the subject or the object of a sentence in detail. They often begin with the relative pro-

nouns who, whom, whose, which, in which, whose, and that, as in the following examples:

> Plato was a philosopher *who studied astronomy, government, and mathematics.*

> The new teacher, *whom you've met before*, will start on Monday.

> In 509 BC, Rome became a republic, *which is a special kind of nation*.

> A republic is a nation *in which power belongs to the citizens.*

> Shakespeare, *whose plays we've read*, was a master of words and images.

> The teacher tutors students *whose math skills are weak.*

> Monks lived in communities *that were called monasteries.*

> Blood cells from a cut form a clot, *which plugs the wound.*

> The Baker's Neighbor is a play *that has been around a long time.*

SUBORDINATE CLAUSES THAT CONTAIN NONFINITE VERBS

The main clause of a sentence always contains a finite verb marked for person (1st, 2nd, 3rd), tense (present, past, future), and number (singular, plural; see Chapter 10). However, subordinate clauses sometimes have a nonfinite verb, which is unmarked for person, tense, and number. These include infinitives, participles, and gerunds.

1. Each of the following complex sentences contains a subordinate clause with an infinitive [INF] clause:

   > John wants *to walk* home after work today.

   > They wanted *to go* to the basketball game.

   > Birds need leaves and twigs *to build* their nests.

   > Rivers, oceans, and forests continue *to change.*

   > With infinitive verbs, the word *to* is sometimes omitted:

   > All I did was *send* him home.

   > Rather than have Ruth *do* it, I'll ask Jimmy.

   > I saw the kitten *chase* the lizard.

2. Nonfinite verbs also include participles [PRT]. Like adjectives, they describe nouns and function like relative clauses. Participles end in -ing, -en, and -ed. Each of the following complex sentences contains a subordinate clause with a participial [PRT] clause:

> *Wearing a new dress,* the princess spoke softly.
>
> *Not easily discouraged,* the basketball team fought its way to victory.
>
> *Buoyed by the good news,* the travelers drove through the night.
>
> *Broken by the baseball,* the window was replaced.

These examples could easily be turned into full-fledged relative clauses:

> The princess, *who was wearing a new dress,* spoke softly.
>
> The basketball team, *which was not easily discouraged,* fought its way to victory.
>
> The travelers, *who were buoyed by the good news,* drove through the night.
>
> The window, *which was broken by the baseball,* was replaced.

3. Nonfinite verbs also include gerunds, which act like nouns and function like nominal clauses. The following complex sentences contain gerundive [GER] clauses:

> *Planting crops in mountainous regions* is often unsuccessful.
>
> *Overusing certain medicines* can cause serious illness.
>
> *Building roads and bridges* provides jobs for many people.
>
> Most people enjoy *going out to dinner and watching a show.*
>
> The man's indigestion resulted from *eating too many spicy foods.*
>
> *Choosing your friends carefully* will bring you much happiness.

When participles or gerunds are used in place of single words (adjectives or nouns), they are *not* considered to be clauses, as in these examples:

The *exhausted* collie swam to shore.

The *broken* toy was repaired.

Swimming is his favorite sport.

Cooking is an enjoyable hobby.

However, when participles occur with other words and act like truncated (reduced) relative clauses, they are considered to be subordinate clauses:

The fence, *broken by the severe windstorm*, was removed.

Martha, *rounding the final curve*, took the lead.

The collie, *exhausted by his rescue effort*, swam to shore.

Similarly, when gerunds occur with other words and act like truncated (reduced) nominal clauses, they are considered to be subordinate clauses:

The lead runner had the job of *setting the pace for the others*.

The Smith family enjoyed *preparing Sunday dinner for the Scouts*.

Arguing against the proposal helped the candidate win the election.

EXERCISES: IDENTIFYING TYPES OF CLAUSES

Exercise 11–1

For the following sets of proverbs, fill in the clause type, using the following codes.

MC = main clause   INF = infinitive clause

REL = relative clause PRT = participial clause

ADV = adverbial clause GER = gerundive clause

NOM = nominal clause

After completing a set, check your answers in the appendix before proceeding to the next set. (Sources: *Category: Proverbs,* http://en.wiki quote.org/wiki/; *Creative proverbs from around the world,* http://creative proverbs.com; Politis, Reich, & Sheldon, 1998; Quotations Page (www.quotationspage.com), Scheffler, 1997; Stewart, 1997; Williams, 2000).

African Proverbs

1. A cutting word is [_____] worse than a bowstring. A cut may heal [_____], but the cut of the tongue does [_____] not.

2. Ashes fly [_____] back into the face of him who throws [_____] them.

3. He who is being carried [_____] does not realize [_____] how far the town is [_____].

4. Quarrels end [_____] but words once spoken never die [_____].

5. Send [_____] a boy where he wants [_____] to go [_____] and you see [_____] his best pace.

6. Smooth seas do not make [_____] skillful sailors.

7. The lion does not turn [_____] around when a small dog barks [_____].

8. Two birds disputed [_____] about a kernel, when a third swooped [_____] down and carried [_____] it off.

9. When a needle falls [_____] into a deep well, many people will look [_____] into the well, but few will be [_____] ready to go [_____] down after it.

10. He who learns [_____] teaches [_____].

Chinese Proverbs

11. A bit of fragrance clings [_____] to the hand that gives [_____] flowers.

12. Even a hare will bite [_____] when it is [_____] cornered.

13. A good fortune may forebode [_____] a bad luck, which may in turn disguise [_____] a good fortune.

14. If you are [_____] patient in a moment of anger, you will escape [_____] a hundred days of sorrow.

15. If you do not study [_____] hard when young, you'll end [___] up bewailing [_____] your failures as you grow up [_____].

16. Learning is [_____] a treasure that will follow [_____] its owner everywhere.

17. Listen [_____] to all, plucking [_____] a feather from every passing goose, but follow [_____] no one absolutely.

18. Make [_____] happy those who are [_____] near, and those who are [_____] far will come [_____].

19. Only when all contribute [_____] their firewood can they build [_____] up a strong fire.

20. To attract [_____] good fortune, spend [_____] a new coin on an old friend, share [_____] an old pleasure with a new friend, and lift [_____] up the heart of a true friend by writing [_____] his name on the wings of a dragon.

Danish Proverbs

21. It is [_____] better to ask [_____] twice than to lose [_____] your way once.

22. He who builds [_____] according [_____] to every man's advice will have [_____] a crooked house.

23. Even a small star shines [_____] in the darkness.

24. A slip of the foot may soon be recovered [_____], but that of the tongue perhaps never.

25. Kind words don't wear [_____] out the tongue.

26. Bad is [_____] never good until worse happens [_____].

27. Let [_____] deeds match [_____] words.

28. Speaking [_____] silence is [_____] better than senseless speech.

29. It is [_____] easy to sit [_____] at the helm in fine weather.

30. A good plan today is [_____] better than a perfect plan tomorrow.

German Proverbs

31. A good conscience is [_____] a soft pillow.

32. A single penny fairly got [_____] is [_____] worth a thousand that are [_____] not.

33. All are [_____] not asleep who have [_____] their eyes shut.

34. Be [_____] silent, or say [_____] something better than silence.

35. Could everything be done [_____] twice, everything would be done [_____] better.

36. If you would have the lamp burn, [_____], you must pour [_____] oil into it.

37. Instead of complaining [_____] that the rosebush is [_____] full of thorns, be [_____] happy that the thorn bush has [_____] roses.

38. It is [_____] better to turn [_____] back than go [_____] astray.

39. It is [_____] not till the cow has lost [_____] her tail, that she discovers [_____] its value.

40. Small undertakings give [_____] great comfort.

Hebrew Proverbs

41. Admission by the defendant is [_____] worth a hundred witnesses.

42. Do not confine [_____] your children to your own learning, for they were born [_____] in another time.

43. Happy is [_____] the generation where the great listen [_____] to the small, for it follows [_____] that in such a generation the small will listen [_____] to the great.

44. Opinions founded [_____] on prejudice are always sustained [_____] with the greatest violence.

45. Promise [_____] little and do [_____] much.

46. Rivalry of scholars advances [_____] wisdom.

47. The kind man feeds [_____] his cat before sitting [_____] down to dinner.

48. Whoever teaches [_____] his son teaches [_____] not only his son but also his son's son, and so on to the end of generations.

49. Who seeks [_____] more than he needs [_____] hinders [_____] himself from enjoying [_____] what he has [_____].

50. Slander slays [_____] three persons: the speaker, the spoken to, and the spoken of.

Irish Proverbs

51. Don't crow [_____] until you're [_____] out of the woods.

52. Many an honest heart beats [_____] under a ragged coat.

53. The thing that is [_____] bought dear is often sold [_____] cheap.

54. Every dog is [_____] bold on its own doorstep.

55. Distant hills look [_____] green.

56. All happy endings are [_____] beginnings as well.

57. Praise [_____] the young and they will blossom [_____].

58. A handful of skill is [_____] better than a bagful of gold.

59. Time is [_____] a great storyteller.

60. It takes [_____] time to build [_____] castles.

Japanese Proverbs

61. A single arrow is easily broken [_____], but not ten in a bundle.

62. If you understand [_____] everything, you must be [_____] misinformed.

63. Laughter cannot bring [_____] back what anger has driven [_____] away.

64. One who smiles [_____] rather than rages [_____] is [_____] always the stronger.

65. We are [_____] no more than candles burning [_____] in the wind.

66. When you're [_____] thirsty, it's [_____] too late to think [_____] about digging [_____] a well.

67. The bamboo that bends [_____] is [_____] stronger than the oak that resists [_____].

68. If money be [_____] not thy servant, it will be [_____] thy master.

69. If you believe [_____] everything you read [_____], better not read [_____].

70. If you want [_____] a thing done well, do [_____] it yourself.

Mexican Proverbs

71. Conversation is [_____] food for the soul.

72. One must learn [_____] how to lose [_____] before learning [_____] how to play [_____].

73. Tell [_____] me who your friends are [_____] and I'll tell [_____] you who you are [_____].

74. It's [_____] not the fault of the mouse, but of the one who offers [_____] him the cheese.

75. In youth we learn [_____], in old age we understand [_____].

76. Money is [_____] a good servant but an evil master.

77. Lions believe [_____] that everyone shares [_____] their state of mind.

78. It is [_____] not enough to know [_____] how to ride [_____]; you must also know [_____] how to fall [_____].

79. He who lives [_____] with hope dies [_____] happy.

80. When the river sounds [_____], it's [_____] because it carries [_____] water.

Russian Proverbs

81. If you travel [_____] more slowly, you will get [_____] farther.

82. A word is [_____] not a sparrow. If it flies [_____] away, you won't catch [_____] it.

83. Not everything that glitters [_____] is [_____] gold.

84. Once you've committed [_____] yourself to move [_____], don't say [_____] you are [_____] not up to it.

85. Any fish is [_____] good if it is [_____] on the hook.

86. All's [_____] well that ends [_____] well.

87. One who sits [_____] between two chairs may easily fall [_____] down.

88. You will reap [_____] what you will sow [_____].

89. We do not care [_____] of what we have [_____], but we cry [_____] when it is [_____] lost.

90. It is [_____] good to be [_____] visiting, but it is [_____] better at home.

Scottish Proverbs

91. A tale never loses [_____] in the telling.

92. Take care [_____] of your pennies and your dollars will take care [_____] of themselves.

93. They that dance [_____] must pay [_____] the fiddler.

94. They that will not be counseled [_____] cannot be helped [_____].

95. What may be [_____] done at any time will be [_____] done at no time.

96. Willful waste makes [_____] woeful want.

97. They that sow [_____] the wind shall reap [_____] the whirlwind.

98. When the cup is [_____] full, carry [_____] it even.

99. Confession is [_____] good for the soul.

100. Get [_____] bait while the tide is [_____] out.

Exercise 11–2

For the following quotations, fill in the clause type, using the following codes.

MC = main clause   INF = infinitive clause

REL = relative clause   PRT = participial clause

ADV = adverbial clause   GER = gerundive clause

NOM = nominal clause

After you complete a set, check your answers in the appendix before proceeding to the next set. (*Sources:* Bachelder, 1965; Benardete, 1961; Burke, 1996; Charlton, 1994; Great Quotations, 1990; Hauser, 2008; McLellan, 1996; Quotable Shakespeare, n.d.; Searls, 2009; Thankful Kids, 2009; Who Said?, 2003).

Set A

1. I took [_____] a speed-reading course and read [_____] *War and Peace* in 20 minutes. It's [_____] about Russia. (Woody Allen)

2. I was [_____] seldom able to see [_____] an opportunity until it had ceased [_____] to be [_____] one. (Mark Twain)

3. I must say [_____] I find [_____] television very educational. The minute somebody turns [_____] it on, I go [_____] to the library and read [_____] a good book. (Groucho Marx)

4. Extemporaneous speaking should be practiced [_____] and cultivated [_____]. It is [_____] the lawyer's avenue to the public. (Abraham Lincoln)

5. Books were [_____] my pass to personal freedom. I learned [_____] to read [_____] at age three, and I soon discovered [_____] there was [_____] a whole world to conquer [_____] that went [_____] beyond our farm in Mississippi. (Oprah Winfrey)

6. Modern cynics and skeptics see [_____] no harm in paying [_____] those to whom they entrust [_____] the minds of their children a smaller wage than is [_____] paid to those to whom they entrust [_____] the care of their plumbing. (John F. Kennedy)

7. It has been said [_____] of the world's history hitherto that might makes [_____] right. It is [_____] for us and for our time to reverse [_____] the maxim and to say [_____] that right makes [_____] might. (Abraham Lincoln)

8. Most of the luxuries, and many of the so-called comforts of life, are [_____] not only not indispensable, but positive hindrances to the elevation of mankind. With respect to luxuries and comforts, the wisest have ever lived [_____] a more simple and meager life than the poor. The ancient philosophers, Chinese, Hindoo, Persian, and Greek, were [_____] a class than which none has been [_____] poorer in outward riches, none so rich in inward. (Henry David Thoreau)

9. Upon the subject of education, not presuming to dictate [_____] any plan or system respecting [_____] it, I can only say [_____] that I view [_____] it as the most important subject which we as a people can be engaged [_____] in. That every man may receive [_____] at least a moderate education, and thereby be [_____] enabled to read [_____] the histories of his own and other countries, by which he may duly appreciate[_____] the value of our free institutions, appears [_____] to be [_____] an object of vital importance. (Abraham Lincoln)

10. I always wanted [_____] to be [_____] somebody, but I should have been [_____]more specific. (Lily Tomlin)

Set B

11. Once they notice [_____] you, they never completely close [_____] the file. (Philip K. Dick).

12. I am [_____] invisible, understand [_____], simply because people refuse [_____] to see [_____] me. (Ralph Ellison)

13. Freedom is [_____] indivisible. (Nelson Mandela)

14. But to live [_____] outside the law, you must be [_____] honest. (Bob Dylan)

15. It ain't [_____] over 'til it's [_____] over. (Yogi Berra)

16. For the spectator even more than for the artist, art is [_____] a habit-forming drug. (Marcel Duchamp)

17. Though I am [_____] in the depths of misery, there is [_____] still calmness, pure harmony and music inside me. (Vincent van Gogh)

18. Never in the field of human conflict was [_____] so much owed [_____] by so many to so few. (Winston Churchill)

19. Time spent [_____] with a cat is [_____] never wasted. (Sydney Hauser)

20. Everybody talks [_____] about people, but nobody ever does [_____] anything about them. (Fran Lebowitz)

Set C

21. I want [_____] to bend [_____] this note, bend [_____] that note, sing [_____] this way, sing [_____] that way, and get [_____] all the feeling, eat [_____] all the good foods, and travel [_____] all over in one day, and you can't do [_____] it. (Billie Holiday)

22. Happy is [_____] the house that shelters [_____] a cat. (Sydney Hauser)

23. If I had [_____] to sum [_____] up the totality of the Woodstock experience, I would say [_____] it was [_____] the first attempt to land [_____] a man on the Earth. (Abbie Hoffman)

24. Never doubt [_____] that a small group of thoughtful, committed people can change [_____] the world. (Margaret Mead)

25. Let [_____] them eat [_____] cake. (Marie-Antoinette)

26. To thine own self be [_____] true, and it must follow [_____], as the night the day, thou canst not then be [_____] false to any man. (William Shakespeare)

27. The future always looks [_____] good in the golden land, because no one remembers [_____] the past. (Joan Didion)

28. In the attitude of silence, the soul finds [_____] the path in a clearer light, and what is [_____] elusive and deceptive resolves [_____] itself into crystal clearness. (Mahatma Gandhi)

29. Half-finished work generally proves [_____] to be [_____] labor lost. (Abraham Lincoln)

30. We have lived [_____] not in proportion to the number of years that we have spent [_____] on the Earth, but in proportion as we have enjoyed [_____]. (Henry David Thoreau)

Set D

31. Nothing so needs [_____] reforming as other people's habits. (Mark Twain)

32. Happiness lies [_____] in the joy of achievement and the thrill of creative effort. (Franklin D. Roosevelt)

33. Brevity is [_____] the soul of wit. (William Shakespeare)

34. Keep [_____] your face to the sunshine and you cannot see [_____] the shadow. (Helen Keller)

35. The time to repair [_____] the roof is [_____] when the sun is shining [_____]. (John F. Kennedy)

36. The only way to get [_____] the best of an argument is [_____] to avoid [_____] it. (Dale Carnegie)

37. California is [_____] a Garden of Eden, a paradise to live [_____] in or see [_____]. (Woody Guthrie)

38. Fair is [_____] foul, and foul is [_____] fair. (William Shakespeare)

39. Be [_____] who you are [_____] and say [_____] what you feel
    [_____]. (Dr. Seuss)

40. All philosophers must soar [_____] with unwearied passion until they
    grasp [_____] the true nature of things as they really are [_____]. (Plato)

Set E

41. The young boy asked [_____], "Why should I become [_____] a
    scholar when I can make [_____] more money in the market place?"
    Plato replied [_____] that, "the pursuit of wisdom and truth is [_____]
    essential to our integrity as human beings."

42. Moving [_____] the ship of state is [_____] a slow process. States are
    [_____] like big tankers. They're [_____] not like speedboats. (Barack
    Obama)

43. Good leadership requires [_____] you to surround [_____] yourself
    with people of diverse perspectives who can disagree [_____] with
    you without fear of retaliation. (Doris Kearns Goodwin)

44. Sometimes leadership is [_____] planting [_____] trees under whose
    shade you'll never sit [_____]. (Jennifer M. Granholm)

45. It takes [_____] 20 years to build [_____] a reputation and five
    minutes to ruin [_____] it. If you think [_____] about that, you'll do
    [_____] things differently. (Warren Buffett)

46. How wonderful it is [_____] that nobody need [_____] wait [_____] a
    single moment before starting [_____] to improve [_____] the world.
    (Anne Frank)

47. Unless someone like you cares [_____] a whole lot, nothing is going
    [_____] to get [_____] better. It's [_____] not. (Dr. Seuss)

48. With every good deed, you are sowing [_____] a seed, though the
    harvest you may not see [_____]. (Anonymous)

49. The more we study [_____] the more we discover [_____] our ignorance. (Percy Bysshe Shelley)

50. My teacher helps [_____] me out a lot and she is [_____] nice to me and she teaches [_____] me about stuff and when I first came [_____] to her classroom, I was [_____] afraid of bugs but now I'm [_____] not. (Krysten, age 8)

Set F

51. Education is [_____] what survives [_____] when what has been learned [_____] has been forgotten [_____]. (B. F. Skinner)

52. My karate teacher can break [_____] 12 bats over his head and 10 bricks with his bare hands. (Billy, age 7)

53. My teacher is [_____] fun and hard-working and never forgets [_____] to take [_____] time to talk [_____] to her students, unlike some teachers who only teach [_____] and never talk [_____]. (Sarah, age 11)

54. The mystic chords of memory, stretching [_____] from every battlefield and patriot grave, to every living heart and hearthstone, all over this broad land, will yet swell [_____] the chorus of the Union, when again touched [_____], as surely they will be [_____], by the better angels of our nature. (Abraham Lincoln; Wilson, 2006, p. 67)

55. I remember [_____] when my second-grade teacher pushed [_____] me and pushed me [_____] to read [_____] and when I finally started [_____] to read [_____], I liked [_____] it so much I couldn't stop [_____]! (Chris, age 8)

56. The art of teaching [_____] is [_____] the art of assisting [_____] discovery. (Mark Van Doren)

57. Human history becomes [_____] more and more a race between education and catastrophe. (H. G. Wells)

58. Leave [_____] it longer on top, so I can have [_____] spikes. My mom wrote [_____] on the form, "no Mohawk," so I can't get [_____] that. (David, age 13)

59. I am [_____] thankful for my dad because he never yells [_____] at me. (Victor, 2nd grade)

60. I'm [_____] thankful that the Ducks are going [_____] to beat [_____] the Beavers. I'm [_____] thankful that I have [_____] clothes to wear [_____] and parents who care [_____] about me. (Frankie, 7th grade)

Exercise 11–3

For the following fable, fill in the clause type, using the following codes.

MC = main clause   INF = infinitive clause

REL = relative clause   PRT = participial clause

ADV = adverbial clause   GER = gerundive clause

NOM = nominal clause

The Lion and the Mouse (Grosset & Dunlap, 1947, pp. 137–138)

A lion was [_____] asleep in his den one day, when a mischievous mouse for no reason at all ran [_____] across the outstretched paw and up the royal nose of the king of beasts, awakening [_____] him from his nap. The mighty beast clapped [_____] his paw upon the now thoroughly frightened little creature and would have made [_____] an end of him.

"Please," squealed [_____] the mouse, "don't kill [_____] me. Forgive [_____] me this time, O King, and I shall never forget [_____] it. A day may come [_____], who knows, when I may do [_____] you a good turn to repay [_____] your kindness." The lion, smiling [_____] at his little prisoner's fright and amused [_____] by the thought that so small a creature ever could be [_____] of assistance to the king of beasts, let [_____] him go [_____].

Not long afterward the lion, while ranging [_____] the forest for his prey, was caught [_____] in the net which the hunters had set [_____] to catch [_____] him. He let [_____] out a roar that echoed [_____] through the forest. Even the mouse heard [_____] it, and recognizing [_____] the voice of his former preserver and friend, ran [_____] to the spot where he lay [_____] tangled in the net of ropes.

"Well, your majesty," said [_____] the mouse, "I know [_____] you did not believe [_____] me once when I said [_____] I would return [_____] a kindness, but here is [_____] my chance." And without further ado he set [_____] to work [_____] to nibble [_____] with his sharp little teeth at the ropes that bound [_____] the lion. Soon the lion was able [_____] to crawl [_____] out of the hunter's snare and be [_____] free.

Application: No act of kindness, no matter how small, is [_____] ever wasted.

Proverb: One good turn deserves [_____] another.

Exercise 11–4. Coding Child and Adolescent Language Samples

The following exercises provide additional practice coding clauses in spoken or written language samples (or excerpts of samples) that were produced by children and adolescents. For each exercise, fill in the blanks using the following codes:

MC = main clause   INF = infinitive clause
REL = relative clause   PRT = participial clause
ADV = adverbial clause   GER = gerundive clause
NOM = nominal clause

#1: *Judy, 11th grade (TLD)* (from the author's files)

General Conversation Task:

1. I'm [_____] a junior.

2. I think [_____] I want [_____] to go [_____] into the elementary educational field.

3. I like [_____] little kids.

4. I'm taking [_____] keyboarding, ITT, which is [_____] international trade and tourism, and a cooking class called [_____] world cooking.

5. And then I'm taking [_____] English.

6. And I have [_____] a worker's experience period where I go [_____] and work [_____] at my job (so).

7. I work [_____] for an insurance company right now.

8. So I work [_____] there doing [_____] the filing.

9. It makes [_____] the car payment.

10. (So we get) so we already have [_____] college credit.

Favorite Game or Sport Task:

1. And there's [_____] foul balls, which means [_____] there's [_____] lines drawn [_____] from the home plate through the first base out to the field like to the fence like 180 feet.

2. And then there's [_____] a line drawn [_____] from the third base line that goes [_____] out.

3. And if the ball goes [_____] past the line to the left in the line not in the playing field, it's [_____] a foul ball.

4. And that's [_____] just a ball.

5. So (it) your count is [_____] still there.

6. And you have [_____] a count when you're [_____] at bat.

7. And then (four balls or yeah) four balls means [_____] you walk [_____].

8. And so when you get [_____] the base automatically, you can't make [_____] an out with that.

9. And then (the base runners) like if you're [_____] on base, you can advance [_____] as soon as the ball leaves [_____] the pitcher's hand.

10. And you can run [_____] the bases until you get [_____] out or until your coach tells [_____] you to stop [_____].

Peer Conflict Resolution Task:

Examiner: What is a good way for Debbie to deal with Melanie?

1. Maybe if there's [_____] a writing part, she can do [_____] the writing part and at least be [_____] there and help [_____] them and try [_____] to say [_____] what she feels [_____] about the whole thing and see [_____] if she has [_____] any advice of what they should do [_____] better.

2. Or (like if just) basically have [_____] a session where they can just talk [_____] and (see what) split [_____] it up into teamwork, working wise.

Examiner: Why is that a good way for Debbie to deal with Melanie?

3. So she doesn't judge [_____] her.

4. Say [_____] she doesn't do [_____] what she's supposed [_____] to do [_____].

5. But if she talks [_____] to her and sees [_____], then maybe they can change [_____] some things.

6. So that will help [_____].

Examiner: What do you think will happen if Debbie does that?

7. Well, she could either say [_____] "no" and ignore [_____] her.

8. Or she could say [_____] "yes."

9. And they could work [_____] the problem out.

10. But if she says [_____] "no," then I guess [_____] she could go [_____] to the teacher and see [_____] what they could do [_____] about it, see [_____] if maybe she could get [_____] another student to help [_____] them or have [_____] more time so the two can just work [_____] on it, Debbie and the other girl.

#2: *Saeda, 2nd grade* (Thankful Kids, 2009)

Expository Essay

I am [_____] thankful for trees because they make [_____] oxygen for me, water because it will make [_____] me not dehydrated, and books because when I read [_____], I can learn [_____] and I love [_____] to read.

#3: *Alex, 3rd grade* (Thankful Kids, 2009)

Expository Essay

These are [_____] some things I am [_____] thankful for. I'm [_____] thankful for my food, my lunch, and everything that is [_____] in it. I'm [_____] glad that it is [_____] a good fruit. I'm [_____] thankful for all the water and milk that we have [_____]. I'm [_____] thankful for my house. My house is [_____] warm and cozy. I love [_____] my house so much. My house is [_____] special. I am [_____] thankful for my school. I'm [_____] so thankful for my teacher. I'm [_____] thankful for all the recess we get [_____]. I'm [_____] thankful for my special book. I'm [_____] so lucky for all these things.

#4: *Kyra, 5th grade* (Thankful Kids, 2009)

Expository Essay

I'm [_____] so thankful for my pets to be [_____] a part of my family. Every single day, I wake up [_____] with warmth on my legs from my dog Toby sleeping [_____] on my legs. When Toby hears [_____] my bus, he will wait [_____] at the door until I come [_____] home. Right when Toby sees [_____] me, he will lick [_____] me until I can't feel [_____] my face and all I can taste [_____] is [_____] slobber. I am [_____] so happy and thankful to have [_____] a dog like Toby.

#5: *Paris, 7th grade* (Thankful Kids, 2009)

Expository Essay

I am [_____] very thankful to have [_____] a mom that can be [_____] around me, even if I don't always want [_____] her around. She comforts [_____] me when I'm [_____] sad or sick. She helps [_____] me through the bad times. She cooks [_____] and provides [_____] for me even if there's [_____] barely anything in the bank. She is [_____] my mother. And her name is [_____] Pam. But don't you wear [_____] it out. That's [_____] my job. I'm [_____] very thankful for a mother that cares [_____].

#6: *Roberto, 8th grade* (Thankful Kids, 2009)

Letter to a Former Teacher

There are [_____] many people in my life for whom I'm [_____] thankful for. But you are [_____] the only person that comes [_____] to mind when I think [_____] of it. Through help and guidance, you are [_____] the one who helped [_____] me through sixth grade. I remember [_____] when you gave [_____] me the Honor Society application sheet. You told [_____] me to get [_____] every teacher to sign [_____] my recommendation sheets and to write [_____] the essay to tell [_____] why I should be [_____] in the Honor Society. You made [_____] sure that I got [_____] my essay done and my recommendation sheets in. You made [_____] sure I was doing [_____] it because you knew [_____] that I would have [_____] a chance to be [_____] in the Honor Society. I truly believe [_____] that without you, I would have never gotten [_____] to where I am [_____] today. I will never forget [_____] the things you did [_____] for me. And that's [_____] why I wanted [_____] to say [_____], "Thank you."

#7: *Emily, 3rd grade (TLD)* (from the author's files)

Narrative Essay: "The Swan"

Once upon a time, there was [_____] a swan. She was going [_____] to have [_____] some babies. But she had never had [_____] babies before. She was [_____] nervous! So she asked [_____] the falcon for some advice. But *she* [the falcon] was asking [_____] that same question. So they went [_____] to look [_____] for someone to help [_____] them. So they asked [_____] the raven for her advice. She said [_____], "Ask [_____] the ostrich. She knows [_____]." They went [_____] to the ostrich. She said [_____] she thought [_____] and thought [_____]. At last, she said [_____], "Why don't you try [_____] laying [_____] on the nest and wait [_____] a while. And they will hatch [_____]. That's [_____] what I would do [_____]." So they went [_____] to their nests and sat [_____] and sat [_____] . And then they said [_____], "I feel [_____] something wiggling." "It must be [_____] the babies," said [_____] the swan and raven. And that was [_____] it. And of course they were [_____] very excited. The end.

#8: Ryan, 5th grade (TLD) (from the author's files)

Expository Essay: The Nature of Friendship

Do you have [_____] a friend? I do [_____]. What do you think [_____] friendship means [_____]? I think [_____] it means [_____] someone you can trust [_____], someone you can depend [_____] on, someone you have [_____] a lot in common with, and somebody who keeps [_____] secrets. Sometimes people feel [_____] lonely and have [_____] no one to talk [_____] to. That can lead [_____] to sadness. That is [_____] some reasons why friendship is [_____] important. Sometimes friendship comforts [_____] you and makes [_____] you feel [_____] less alone. Me and my friends like [_____] to play [_____] lots and lots of video games together. Some advice for good friendship is [_____] to not annoy [_____] the person, be [_____] nice to the person. Do not tell [_____] secrets that they have told [_____] you.

#9: Mark, 8th grade (TLD) (from the author's files)

Expository Essay: The Nature of Friendship

Friendship is [_____] basically an understanding between two people who share [_____] common interests or beliefs. Friendship is

[_____] about being [_____] able to trust [_____] that person and being
[_____] able to spend [_____] time with them. Friendship is [_____]
important to people because it gives [_____] them a chance to do [_____]
things that they like [_____] with someone they enjoy [_____] spending
[_____] time with. Having [_____] friends makes [_____] life more
enjoyable because you have [_____] someone you can talk [_____] to
and that you like [_____] to do [_____] things with. Friends do [_____] all
kinds of things together from going [_____] on hikes to going [_____] to
the movies. Friends can talk [_____] to each other and go [_____] places
together. People who generally become [_____] friends are [_____] those
who have [_____] common interests. If someone had [_____] completely
different opinions about what is [_____] fun to do [_____] than someone
else, then they probably won't become [_____] very good friends. The
kinds of things that can harm [_____] a friendship are [_____] things like
arguing and fighting. If you intentionally do [_____] something that you
know [_____] they won't like [_____], it will damage [_____] a friendship.
A way to maintain [_____] a friendship is [_____] to continually spend
[_____] time with them. That way you can still talk [_____] to each other
even if they live [_____] a long ways away. That can help [_____] people
remain [_____] friends. There are [_____] always ways to maintain [_____]
friendships. Sometimes it is [_____] just hard to figure [_____] out how.

#10: *Willow, 8th grade* (Teachers Need to Be Healthy, 2009)

Letter to the Editor (Persuasive Essay)

We think [_____] that the ban of junk foods in schools should
include [_____] teachers. Sodas and other junk foods are [_____] just
as unhealthy for teachers as they are [_____] for students. The teachers
need [_____] to set [_____] a good example for the students. If students
see [_____] that the ban on junk food includes [_____] teachers as well
as themselves, they might be [_____] more willing to go [_____] along
with the ban. To have [_____] a mind and body that functions [_____] the
best they can [_____], you need [_____] to eat [_____] the proper amount

of nutrients. You do not get [_____] these nutrients from junk foods and soda. Because of this, you do not function [_____] as well as you could [_____]. We think [_____] it is [_____] important for teachers to have [_____] healthy bodies and minds, so that they will teach [_____] the students better than otherwise. If teachers eat or drink [_____] junk food or soda, they will not teach [_____] as well.

If the teachers really cannot live [_____] without the junk food, they can very easily just eat [_____] it at their homes. It should not be [_____] that hard for them to wait [_____] the seven or eight hours that their jobs take [_____] up to eat [_____] junk food if they need [_____] it that badly. After all, students can [_____].

#11: Trevor, 5th grade (TLD) (from the author's files)

Persuasive Essay: The Circus Controversy

I think [_____] it is [_____] a bad idea to have [_____] animals in the circus because animals should be [_____] free to do [_____] what they want [_____]. They're [_____] stuck in small cages. So there is [_____] barely enough room to get [_____] their adequate exercise. People don't like [_____] to be [_____] imprisoned. So we should let [_____] them go [_____]. Then they won't be [_____] forced to do [_____] tricks. I think [_____] it is [_____] cruel to train [_____] animals to do [_____] a trick because if they don't do [_____] it right, the trainers will hit [_____] them. These are [_____] the reasons why I think [_____] circuses should not be [_____] allowed. For the animals' sake.

#12: Carl, 11th grade (TLD) (from the author's files)

Persuasive Essay: The Circus Controversy

A common controversy is [_____] often whether or not circuses are [_____] good or bad for the community. I like [_____] the clowns because often times they are [_____] also animal trainers. However, there is [_____] a downside to all these beneficial factors. Frequently, the animals are [_____] underfed and are kept [_____] in small cages. This alone infuriates [_____] animal enthusiasts everywhere. Circuses can be [_____] cruel to animals. Therefore, they should be closed [_____] down. If animals feel [_____] threatened, they could be [_____] dangerous when they fight [_____] back. What I believe [_____] is [_____] that a circus could hire [_____] more people and have them go [_____] to clown school. Everybody likes [_____] clowns, right? The hardest part of this would be [_____] training [_____] all those clowns. Still, with a little creativity and some ingenuity, I think [_____] a clown school could be [_____] possible. Overall, I think [_____] animals should not be [_____] in circuses.

CHAPTER 12

Types of Sentences

A sentence is a grammatical construction that can stand by itself and make sense (Crystal, 1996). By definition, every sentence contains a subject and a main verb (finite verb) and expresses a complete thought. There are four basic types of sentences: *simple, complex, compound,* and *compound-complex.*

A simple sentence consists of one main clause (e.g., a duckbill platypus *lays* eggs; it is a mammal; there was a tornado watch). A complex sentence, however, contains one or more subordinate clauses in addition to the main clause (e.g., because the duckbill platypus *produces* milk for its young, scientists *call* it a mammal.) A sentence that contains an infinitive verb in addition to a main clause is also complex:

Because of the tornado watch, the teachers required all students *to stay* inside.

The students and their teachers wanted *to go* home.

To prepare for the tornado, families stored dry foods.

Sentences that contain participles (that act like truncated relative clauses) and gerunds (that act like truncated nominal clauses), in addition to a main clause, also are complex:

Complaining [PRT] about the service, Mary wrote [MC] a letter to the manager.

Building [GER] strong customer relationships was [MC] the manager's primary goal.

A compound sentence contains at least two main clauses that are joined by coordinate conjunctions that include *but*, *and*, *so*, and *or*:

Ice cream contains lots of fat *but* it sure tastes good!

Cherries are fruit *and* artichokes are flowers.

We enjoy cakes *so* we bake them every week.

Fluffy will stay home *or* he will go to the park.

Compound sentences with ellipsis: Sometimes a compound sentence will delete one of the subjects, usually the second one, because it is redundant. This is called ellipsis. In the following sentence, the subject of the second main clause, *they*, is deleted:

The family packed [MC] up their car and drove [MC] to the mountains.

A *compound-complex* sentence contains at least two main clauses and one or more subordinate clauses:

Today, the major environmental concern *is* [MC] global warming, and many scientists *believe* [MC] that excess carbon dioxide *is raising* [NOM] the temperature of the atmosphere.

ACTIVE VERSUS PASSIVE SENTENCES

It is important to distinguish between sentences in the active versus the passive voice. Sentences in the active voice express ideas in a direct and straightforward manner, with the subject clearly stating who performed the main action of the sentence. The following sentences are in the active voice:

John kicked the football.

Mary wrote a letter.

Herman cut the birthday cake.

I expected that Jim would be late.

In contrast, sentences in the passive voice express ideas in an indirect, wordy, and sometimes confusing manner, as in the following examples:

The football was kicked by John.

The letter was written by Mary.

The birthday cake was cut by Herman.

It was expected (by me) that Jim would be late.

Most of the time, the active voice is preferred because it expresses ideas more efficiently. However, sometimes the passive voice is desired when the speaker or writer is attempting to avoid blaming someone for an undesirable act or even to avoid taking responsibility for such an act, for example:

Mistakes were made (by the president of the company who actually knew better)

A motorcycle was parked illegally (by its owner who was late for work)

The house was left unlocked (by its occupant who was tired and distracted)

When coding clauses in sentences that are in the passive voice, it is important to remember that the main verb is still the same verb as in the active voice, and that the code would be placed immediately after that verb, as in these examples:

Mistakes were made [MC] (by the president of the company).

The president of the company made [MC] mistakes.

The motorcycle was parked [MC] illegally (by the owner).

The owner parked [MC] the motorcycle illegally.

The house was left [MC] unlocked (by its occupant).

The occupant left [MC] the house unlocked.

It was expected [MC] that Jim would be [NOM] late.

I expected [MC] that Jim would be [NOM] late.

SUBJECTLESS SENTENCES: COMMAND AND ELLIPSIS

Although every sentence has a subject, command sentences (or imperatives) do not explicitly state the subject, which is understood by the listener. Command sentences commonly occur when someone is giving directions (e.g., eat your soup; be patient; try your best.) In the following paragraph, all sentences except one ("Sauce should be fairly thick.") are commands, and the subject is "you." The finite verbs have been italicized:

Soak mushrooms in warm water for 30 minutes. *Squeeze* dry and *cut* into thin strips. In a large nonstick frying pan, *heat* oil and gently *sauté* the chicken. *Add* garlic and onion. *Discard* garlic as it *begins* to brown. *Continue* cooking until onion *is* limp. *Add* remaining ingredients. *Season* with salt and pepper if desired. *Simmer* 30 minutes, or until chicken *is* tender. Sauce *should be* fairly thick. *Add* water to thin if necessary (Oliva-Rasbach & Schmidt, 1994, p. 364).

Sentences with ellipsis also omit the subject, as in the following examples:

Wish you were here.

Had a great time yesterday.

Told you so.

Looks like rain today.

Want a sandwich?

Hafta go now.

For the preceding sentences, respectively, the subjects are I, I, I, it, you, and I. Ellipsis also can occur when answering a question:

Q: Do you like baseball?

A: Depends on who's playing.

Q: What else happened at the party?

A: Can't remember.

Q: Where'd you go?

A: To the track meet.

Q: Who shall help bake this bread?

A: Don't look at me!

SENTENCE FRAGMENTS

Sentence fragments do not meet the definition of a sentence because they lack a subject and/or a main verb. However, they are acceptable in spoken and written contexts when they make a statement, express meaning, function as if they were complete, and are free of grammatical errors, as with the following examples:

And now for the star of our show . . . Bob Hope!

One for all and all for one. (English proverb)

Far from the eye, far from the heart. (Maltese proverb)

To sleep . . . perchance to dream. (Shakespeare)

Sentence fragments also occur in the context of notes such as those presented in field guides. In the following examples of sentence fragments, note the many adjectives used to describe these native birds of Oregon (Tekiela, 2001):

Brewer's blackbird: An *overall grayish brown* bird (female)

Great Horned owl: A *robust brown "horned"* owl with *bright yellow* eyes and *V-shaped white* bib (male)

Northern pintail: A *slender, elegant* duck with a *brown* head, *white* neck, *gray* body, and extremely *long, narrow, black* tail (male); *mottled brown* body with a *paler* head and neck, *long* tail, *gray* bill (female)

Red-winged blackbird: Jet *black* bird with *red* and *yellow* patches on *upper* wings (male); heavily *streaked brown* bird with *white* eyebrows (female)

Another type of sentence fragment is one in which a subordinate clause occurs in isolation:

When I am fit

However hard we tried

So that I arrived with no fuss, never a minute too soon or too late

Sometimes this type of fragment occurs in natural communication to answer a question or to make a comment. However, to turn them into complete sentences, they must be attached to a main clause as in the following examples (Bannister, 2004):

When I am fit, my running feels effortless.

However hard we tried, it did not seem possible to meet our target of 60 seconds.

They often drove me to athletics meetings so that I arrived with no fuss, never a minute too soon or too late.

HIERARCHICAL COMPLEXITY

Complex sentences often contain more than one subordinate clause. When one subordinate clause is embedded into another subordinate clause, which is embedded into the main clause, a complex hierarchy of clauses occurs (Quirk & Greenbaum, 1973; Scott, 2009). This can be seen in the following sentence:

I think [MC] you will succeed [NOM] if you try [ADV].

With this sentence, the ADV is embedded into the NOM, which is embedded into the MC. With these types of sentences, it is possible to count the levels of embedding that occur. The following sentence contains only one subordinate clause:

> Earthworms are [MC] shredders that can break [REL] large pieces of dead material into smaller pieces.

Because it has only one subordinate clause, the sentence has only one level of embedding (or complexity); the relative clause modifies the noun, *shredders*. In contrast, the following sentence has two levels of embedding, in which the second relative clause modifies the second instance of the noun *pieces*.

> Earthworms are [MC] shredders
>
>> that can break [REL] large pieces of dead material into smaller pieces,
>>
>>> which are [REL] processed by fungi and bacteria

In determining levels of embedding, all verbs in a sentence represent a clause, at least in the deep structure of the sentence. Now consider a quote from Oprah Winfrey:

> Books were [MC] my pass to personal freedom. I learned [MC] to read [INF] at age three, and I soon discovered [MC] there was [NOM] a whole world to conquer [INF] that went [REL] beyond our farm in Mississippi.

The first sentence does not contain any embedding; it is a simple sentence. However, the second sentence, which is compound-complex, contains two levels of embedding:

> I learned
>
>> to read at age three, (level one)
>
> and I soon discovered
>
>> there was a whole world (level one)
>>
>>> to conquer (level two)
>>>
>>> that went beyond our farm in Mississippi (level two)

For another interesting example, consider the following complex sentence:

> If you are complaining [ADV] about a service you received [REL], describe [MC] the service and who performed [NOM] it.

How many levels of embedding do you think it has? To determine this, answer the following questions:

1. What is the main clause? (describe the service)*

2. What nominal clause completes it? (and who performed it)**

3. What adverbial clause introduces the main clause? (if you are complaining about a service)

4. What relative clause modifies the adverbial clause? (you received)

In this sentence, the main clause has two subordinate clauses, the adverbial and the nominal, which are on equal footing. Together, they create one level of complexity. However, the adverbial clause is modified by a relative clause. This adds another level of complexity, so the entire sentence has two levels of embedding.

For an even more interesting example, consider the following complex sentence of 44 words, written by Henry David Thoreau (2004, p. 88):

I went [MC] to the woods because I wished [ADV] to live [INF] deliberately, to front [INF] only the essential facts of life, and see [INF] if I could not learn [NOM] what it had [NOM] to teach [INF], and not, when I came [ADV] to die [INF], discover [INF] that I had not lived [NOM].

I went to the woods

    because I wished (level one)

        to live deliberately (level two)

        to front only the essential facts of life (level two)

        and see (level two)

            if I could not learn (level three)

                what it had (level four)

                    to teach (level five)

            and not, when I came (level three)

                to die (level four)

        discover (level two)

            that I had not lived (level three)

---

*Note that the subject of this imperative main clause is the unstated *you*.

**Note that the metalinguistic verb describe calls for a nominal clause.

EXERCISES: IDENTIFYING TYPES OF SENTENCES

Exercise 12–1

For each quotation, indicate whether the sentence is:

A. Simple   C. Compound

B. Complex   D. Compound-complex

1. _____ All philosophers must soar with unwearied passion until they grasp the true nature of things as they really are. (Plato)

2. _____ Education is not filling a pail but the lighting of a fire. (William Butler Yeats)

3. _____ If you bungle raising your children, I don't think whatever else you do well matters very much. (Jacqueline Kennedy Onassis)

4. _____ A little learning is a dangerous thing. (Alexander Pope)

5. _____ Never give up and never give in. (Hubert H. Humphrey)

6. _____ Life is a festival only to the wise. (Ralph Waldo Emerson)

7. _____ No one can make you feel inferior without your consent. (Eleanor Roosevelt)

8. _____ To talk in public, to think in solitude, to read and to hear, to inquire and answer inquiries, is the business of the scholar. (Samuel Johnson)

9. _____ My teacher is special because she never yells at me. (Rebecca, age 8)

10. _____ There's something about taking a plow and breaking new ground. (Ken Kesey)

11. _____ The more we study, the more we discover our ignorance. (Percy Bysshe Shelley)

12. _____ My teacher helps me out a lot and she is nice to me and she teaches me about stuff and when I first came to her classroom, I was afraid of bugs but now I'm not. (Krysten, age 8)

13. _____ Education is what survives when what has been learned has been forgotten. (B. F. Skinner)

14. _____ My karate teacher can break 12 bats over his head and 10 bricks with his bare hands. (Billy, age 7)

15. _____ My teacher is fun and hard-working and never forgets to take time to talk to her students, unlike some teachers who only teach and never talk. (Sarah, age 11)

16. _____ Mix with your sage counsels some brief folly. (Cicero)

17. _____ I remember when my second-grade teacher pushed me and pushed me to read and when I finally started to read, I liked it so much I couldn't stop! (Chris, age 8)

18. _____ The art of teaching is the art of assisting discovery. (Mark Van Doren)

19. _____ Leave it longer on top, so I can have spikes. (David, age 13)

20. _____ My mom wrote on the form, "no Mohawk," so I can't get that. (David, age 13)

Exercise 12–2. Hierarchical Complexity

For each of the following sentences, indicate the number of levels of embedding it contains. Begin by coding each sentence for each type of clause it contains:

MC = main clause   INF = infinitive clause
REL = relative clause   PRT = participial clause
ADV = adverbial clause   GER = gerundive clause
NOM = nominal clause

1. Even if you're [_____] on the right track, you'll get run [_____] over if you just sit [_____] there.   Levels: _____.

2. With every good deed, you are sowing [_____] a seed, though the harvest you may not see [_____].   Levels: _____.

3. Use [_____] a small paintbrush and a paper cup with the smaller beetles because you can damage [_____] them if you pick [_____] them up in your hand.   Levels: _____.

4. Jason's little sister Amanda has [_____] an ear infection for which her pediatrician prescribed [_____] a liquid antibiotic that must be kept [_____] refrigerated.   Levels: _____.

5. Every miler knows [_____], in the way a sailor knows [_____] the middle of the ocean, that it is [_____] not the first lap but the third that is [_____] farthest from the finish line. (Parker, 2009, p. 246) Levels: _____.

6. As Jim and I went [_____] over to see [_____] what was going [_____] on, someone crawled [_____] out of the closet. (Boy, age 13) Levels: _____.

7. Before you take [_____] a piece, like if there was [_____] a rook right here, you kind of make [_____] sure because there is [_____] a strategy that you can do [_____] to try [_____] to get [_____] a king in checkmate with two rooks. (Boy, age 11)   Levels: _____.

8. I hated [_____] him on sight and sound and would be [_____] about to put [_____] my dog whistle to my lips and blow [_____] him off the face of Christmas when suddenly he, with a violet wink, put [_____] *his* whistle to *his* lips and blew [_____] so stridently, so high, so exquisitely loud, that gobbling faces, their cheeks bulged [_____] with goose, would press [_____] against their tinseled windows, the whole length of the white echoing street. (Thomas, 1954, p. 22) Levels: _____.

Exercise 12–3

Code the following sentences. Then rewrite each sentence in the active voice and code it again.

1. It was promised [_____] by Mozart that the duets would be completed [_____] soon.

   Active: _____

2. The missing duets, which had been misplaced [_____] by Frederick, were presented [_____] by Mozart to his friend Joseph Haydn.

   Active: _____

3. It was known [_____] by all patrons that a symphony could be written [_____] by Mozart in minutes.

   Active: _____

4. An amazing tonal richness was achieved [_____] by the string quartet, which was led [_____] by a new cellist from Philadelphia.

   Active: _____

5. The miniature trio for three strings was created [_____] by the new composer who was paid [_____] handsomely by the king's court.

   Active: _____

6. The young musician was supported [_____] by a generous scholarship funded [_____] by a wealthy elderly patron, to attend [_____] the Juilliard School of Music.

   Active: _____

7. The composer's status of nobility was implied [_____] by the "von" inserted [_____] before his last name, which was preferred [_____] by some over the plainer "Ernst Dohnanyi."

   Active: _____

8. The flute quartet was performed [_____] by four young musicians who had been hired [_____] by a royal family to educate [_____] its children in the finer things in life.

   Active: _____

9. A dramatic conclusion to the Christmas play was anticipated [_____] by members of the audience, many of whom had been coerced [_____] into attending [_____] the performance.

   Active: _____

10. The rock concert, sold out [_____] for months, had to be cancelled [_____] by the vendor because the band's lead singer had been delayed [_____] by inclement weather in Chicago.

    Active: _____

CHAPTER 13

Units of Measurement

*T*his chapter describes some units of measurement that are often used when examining spoken and written language samples. They include the communication unit (C-unit), the terminable unit (T-unit), clausal density (CD), and mean length of utterance (MLU). Issues concerning maze behavior and what constitutes a word are also discussed.

C-UNITS AND T-UNITS

A C-unit or T-unit consists of one main clause and any attached subordinate clauses (Hunt, 1970). C-units, unlike T-units, also may include answers to questions that are incomplete sentences (Loban, 1976). In general, C-units are used when examining spoken language, and T-units are used when examining written language. The following sentences are examples of C-units and T-units:

Cats have been kept as domestic animals for thousands of years.

There are undoubtedly many reasons for the cat's popularity.

Many cat lovers like to attribute it to the cat's personality and beauty.

Cats have many advantages when it comes to choosing a household pet.

When a sentence contains two or more main clauses—each with its own stated subject—it is broken into two or more C-units (or T-units), as shown by the slash (/) in the following examples:

Cats require less care and attention than many other pets, while providing excellent companionship, love, and loyalty / but a cat's love has to be earned /

Cats can become attached to their home territory / and most dislike travel /

With any adult cat, you should remember that some time may be required for it to become attached to its new owner and home / and if allowed outside, it may try to return to its old home or neighborhood / (Wright & Walters, 1980).

However, sometimes a sentence will contain a second main clause whose subject is the same as that of the first main clause but has been deleted via ellipsis. In such cases, the entire sentence is considered to be one C-unit (or T-unit) that contains two coordinated main clauses, as in the following example in which the subject of both clauses is *people*:

Many people moved [MC] to America and entered [MC] at Ellis Island.

MEAN LENGTH OF C-UNIT AND MEAN LENGTH OF T-UNIT

Mean Length of C-unit (MLCU) and Mean Length of T-unit (MLTU) are general indices of syntactic development (Hunt, 1970; Loban, 1976). To calculate MLCU or MLTU, the total number of words produced in a sample is summed and then divided by the total number of C-units or T-units it contains. For example, if a sample contains 250 words and 15 C-units, MLCU = 16.67 words. Alternatively, if the sample contains 360 words and 40 T-units, MLTU = 9.0 words.

In addition to reporting MLCU or MLTU, it is useful to report the total number of words and C-units or T-units contained in a sample. Each of these measures can serve as an index of language productivity (Nippold, 2009). Often, the speech-language pathologist will notice that an adolescent talks more (e.g., produces more words and C-units) about certain topics and less about others, a pattern that could stem from many factors such knowledge of the topic, interest in the topic, and motivation to talk about it. With further investigation of underlying factors, the speech-language pathologist may be able to use that information to design an intervention program that encourages the adolescent to tap into his or her language competencies more fully.

Counting Words

When counting words in a language sample, questions often arise about what constitutes a word. For example, is *Miss Virginia Finley* one, two, or three words? What about contractions such as doesn't, wouldn't, and don't? Are they one or two words each? And what about catenatives such as gonna, lemme, and hafta? When counting words, the following guidelines will help the speech-language pathologist decide what constitutes a word:

1. Proper names are one word even when their spelling suggests otherwise. For example, the following proper names are each one word: Mrs. Jones, David Tompkins, Home Town Buffet, Stratford-Upon-Avon, Smoke-N-Hot Coffee. To ensure that SALT counts each of these names as one word, insert the underscore space (_) between each part with no spaces (e.g., Mrs._Jones, David_Tompkins, Home_Town_Buffet, Stratford_Upon_Avon, Smoke_N_ Hot_Coffee).

2. Compound and hyphenated words are one word (e.g., baseball, mid-valley).

3. Interjections are one word (e.g., Oh! OK! Shh! Ugh! Whew!).

4. Indefinite pronouns are one word (e.g., anybody, somebody, everyone, something).

5. Contractions are two words (e.g., shouldn't, won't, couldn't, let's, we're). To ensure that SALT counts them as two words, insert a space between them, for example: should n't, wo n't, could n't, let 's, we 're.

6. Catenatives are two words (e.g., hafta (have to), sorta (sort of), kinda (kind of)). To ensure that SALT counts them as two words, insert a space between them, for example: haf ta, sor ta, kin da.

7. Fillers such as *um*, *uh*, and *er* are not counted as words, but are mazes.

Ignoring Mazes

Maze behavior consists of false starts, hesitations, and revisions that do not contribute to the clear expression of an idea. When mazes occur in a spoken language sample, they are disregarded. Thus, when transcribing a language sample, all verbalizations that constitute mazes are enclosed in parentheses so that what is left over expresses a coherent idea and is presumed to be the speaker's final formulation. For example, the maze behavior in the following utterances has been parenthesized:

> (The only other thing . . . um . . . uh . . . well, what I mean is) the only thing left to do is to clean up this mess!

When calculating MLCU or MLTU, words in parentheses are not counted. For example, after parenthesizing all mazes, the following sentence would be a 14-word C-unit:

> His dog ran after him (and so . . . uh . . . and . . . and the the), got in the jeep, and rode (it in a) around with him.

Here is another example of how to handle maze behavior in an 11-year-old girl:

> I like Uno. It's kind of challenging. (um . . . all right . . . need about) you can play it with two players or more. You deal out your cards. And I think you get five cards per person. And you look at your cards. And (you flip over it) you have a stack of cards. And you flip over the first card. And (you try to) if you have the card (you have) you lay down the color.

CLAUSAL DENSITY

During adolescence, sentences become longer because they contain a greater number of subordinate clauses, which often are embedded within other subordinate clauses. This phenomenon, which builds hierarchical complexity, increases the density of a sentence. To capture this aspect of development, a metric called *clausal density* is reported. Clausal density is calculated by summing all main and subordinate clauses in a sample and dividing by the total number of C-units (or T-units) produced (Hunt, 1970; Loban, 1976). Following is an example from a hypothetical language sample:

Total main clauses = 52

Total subordinate clauses = 37 (11 = relative; 16 = adverbial; 10 = nominal)

Total clauses (main and subordinate) = 89

Total C-units = 52

Clausal density = 1.71 (89/52 = 1.71)

MEAN LENGTH OF UTTERANCE

Mean length of utterance (MLU) also is used to measure syntactic development in school-age children and adolescents and is used for either spoken or written language samples (e.g., Miller, 2009). When calculating MLU, an utterance may consist of a full sentence as well as a shorter production. To determine MLU, the total number of words produced in a sample is divided by the total number of utterances produced.

MLU is based on all utterances contained in the sample with the exception of mazes (false starts, hesitations, repetitions, revisions). This would include fragments as well as complete sentences. Generally, when calculating MLU, compound sentences are broken into two or more sentences, each with their own associated subordinate clauses. However, if the second coordinated clause has an understood subject that is coreferential with the subject of the first clause and has been deleted via ellipsis, then both clauses are combined into one utterance. For example, the following sentence is one utterance:

The bear wanted her cub to be safe and nudged her into the cave.

ANALYZING A SAMPLE OF WRITTEN LANGUAGE USING SALT

To review the principles discussed in this chapter, examine the following passage, an excerpt from the menu at Antoine's Restaurant in New Orleans, Louisiana (2009). The passage has been broken into T-units and coded for the use of main and subordinate clauses. There are 159 total words and 12 T-units. Therefore, MLTU = 13.25 words. In addition, the passage contains 12 main clauses and 6 subordinate clauses (ADV = 3; INF = 2; REL = 1), for a total of 18 clauses. Therefore, clausal density = 1.5.

There is [MC] only one Antoine's.

It has become [MC] as much a part of New_Orleans as Jackson_Square and Saint_Louis_Cathedral, a restaurant that has been operated [REL] continuously by the same family since 1840.

That is [MC] now over 169 years.

Antoine's has seen [MC] the history of New_Orleans through the Civil_War, World_Wars_I_and_II, the Great_Depression, epidemics, and storms.

It all started [MC] when Antoine_Alciatore arrived [ADV] here from Marseilles, France, in 1840, and became [ADV] immediately a culinary notable.

He was [MC] 16 years old.

Young Antoine had been apprenticed [MC], since the age of eight, to the Great French Chef, Coffient, of the Hotel_de_Noailles in Marseilles.

His parents' wavering fortunes as cloth merchants required [MC] that the young boy learn [INF] a trade and help [INF] the family himself.

By the time he left [ADV] France, Antoine had served [MC] kings and royalty and the aristocracy of that country.

But the voice of opportunity in the new America cried [MC] louder than all else.

He followed [MC] that call.

And it took [MC] him to New_Orleans.

EXERCISES: UNITS OF MEASUREMENT

Exercise 13–1. Identifying T-units

For each of the following paragraphs, indicate with a slash (/) the end of each T-unit:

1. Once Oregon was thought to be immune to earthquakes; today, we know that we have them in three different flavors—devastating subduction earthquakes like the 1700 catastrophe, deep intraplate earthquakes like the Puget_Sound temblors of 1949 and 2001, and sharp local jolts like the Spring_Break_Quake of 1993 (Sullivan, 2008, p. 67).

   > How many T-units are contained in this paragraph? How many words did Sullivan use?

   > What is Sullivan's MLTU?

   > How many of Sullivan's T-units are complex sentences?

2. Beatrix_Potter was a Londoner, born there in 1866 but her family had connections with Lancashire cotton, and she spent her holidays from the age of 16 in the Lake_District, in rented, but rather grand houses, round Windermere and Derwentwater her parents were genteel, upper middle class Edwardians and she was educated at home and expected to devote her life to her parents or get married she found an outlet for artistic talents in drawing and painting "little books for children" and encouraged by the family's Lakeland friend, Canon_Rawnsley, her first book, *Peter_Rabbit*, was published in 1901 (Davies, 1989, p. 179).

   > How many T-units are contained in this paragraph? How many words did Davies use?

   > What is Davies' MLTU?

   > How many T-units are complex sentences?

3. I have become a little more skillful in guessing right explanations and in devising experimental tests but this may probably be the

result of mere practice, and of a larger store of knowledge I have as much difficulty as ever in expressing myself clearly and concisely and this difficulty has caused me a very great loss of time but it has had the compensating advantage of forcing me to think long and intently about every sentence and thus I have been often led to see errors in reasoning and in my own observations or those of others (Charles Darwin, 1958, pp. 136–137)

How many T-units are contained in this paragraph?

How many words did Darwin use?

What is Darwin's MLTU?

How many of Darwin's T-units are complex sentences?

4. Some birds, such as most eagles, hawks, ospreys, falcons, and vultures, migrate during the day larger birds can hold more body fat, go longer without eating, and take longer to migrate these birds glide along on rising columns of warm air, called thermals, which hold them aloft while they slowly make their way north or south they generally rest at night and hunt early in the morning before the sun has a chance to warm up the land and create good soaring conditions birds migrating during the day use a combination of landforms, rivers, and the rising and setting sun to guide them in the right direction (Tekiela, 2001, p. xv)

How many T-units are contained in this paragraph?

How many words did Tekiela use?

What is Tekiela's MLTU?

How many of Tekiela's T-units are complex sentences?

5. In the morning I watched the geese from the door through the mist, sailing in the middle of the pond, fifty rods off, so large and tumultuous that Walden appeared like an artificial pond for their amusement but when I stood on the shore they at once rose up with a great flapping of wings at the signal of their commander, and when they had got into rank circled about over my head,

twenty_nine of them, and then steered straight to Canada, with a regular *honk* from the leader at intervals, trusting to break their fast in muddier pools a "plump" of ducks rose at the same time and took the route to the north in the wake of their noisier cousins (Thoreau, 2004, pp. 301–302)

> How many T-units are contained in this paragraph?
>
> How many words did Thoreau use?
>
> What is Thoreau's MLTU?
>
> How many of Thoreau's T-units are complex sentences?

6. Upon the subject of education, not presuming to dictate any plan or system respecting it, I can only say that I view it as the most important subject which we as a people can be engaged in that every man may receive at least a moderate education, and thereby be enabled to read the histories of his own and other countries, by which he may duly appreciate the value of our free institutions, appears to be an object of vital importance (Abraham Lincoln, cited by Bachelder, 1965, p. 7)

> How many T-units are contained in this paragraph?
>
> How many words did Lincoln use?
>
> What is Lincoln's MLTU?
>
> How many of Lincoln's T-units are complex sentences?

7. I have been the whole day without eating and the whole night without sleeping, occupied with thinking it was no use the better plan is to learn learning without thought is labor lost and thought without learning is perilous (Confucius, 6th century B.C., Peter Pauper Press, 1963, p. 42)

> How many T-units are contained in this paragraph?
>
> How many words did Confucius use?
>
> What is Confucius's MLTU?
>
> How many of Confucius's T-units are complex sentences?

8. The critical habit of thought, if usual in a society, will pervade all its mores, because it is a way of taking up the problems of life men educated in it cannot be stampeded by stump orators and are never deceived by dithyrambic oratory they are slow to believe they can hold things as possible or probable in all degrees, without certainty and without pain they can wait for evidence and weigh evidence, uninfluenced by the emphasis or confidence with which assertions are made on one side or the other they can resist appeals to their dearest prejudices and all kinds of cajolery education in the critical faculty is the only education of which it can be truly said that it makes good citizens (William Graham Sumner, 1906, p. 633)

> How many T-units are contained in this paragraph?
>
> How many words did Sumner use?
>
> What is Sumner's MLTU?
>
> How many of Sumner's T-units are complex sentences?

9. Inside England, as we have seen, one form of the language, basically an East_Midland dialect, became accepted as a literary standard in the late Middle_Ages and with this went a prestige accent based on that of the court in Westminster this does not mean that dialect differences disappeared in England Standard_English was the language of a small minority most speakers used a nonstandard form of the language and in each area there was a speech hierarchy corresponding to the class hierarchy, differing from Standard_English not only in accent but also in grammar and vocabulary the higher the socioeconomic level of the speakers, the nearer their speech was likely to be to Standard_English, though the degree of formality of the situation also influenced the level of speech used (Barber, 1993, p. 232).

> How many T-units are contained in this paragraph?
>
> How many words did Barber use?
>
> What is Barber's MLTU?
>
> How many of Barber's T-units are complex sentences?

10. We are a nation of Christians and Muslims, Jews, and Hindus, and non_believers we are shaped by every language and culture, drawn from every end of this Earth and because we have tasted the bitter swill of civil war and segregation, and emerged from that dark chapter stronger and more united, we cannot help but believe that the old hatreds shall someday pass, that the lines of tribe shall soon dissolve, that as the world grows smaller, our common humanity shall reveal itself, and that America must play its role in ushering in a new era of peace (Barack Obama, 2009)

> How many T-units are contained in this paragraph?
>
> How many words did Obama use?
>
> What is Obama's MLTU?
>
> How many of Obama's T-units are complex sentences?

Exercise 13–2. Identifying Maze Behavior in Adolescent Speakers

The utterances here were produced by adolescents who were talking about sports and conflicts. For each utterance, use parentheses to enclose the maze behavior. What is left over should be a clean, coherent utterance, presumably the speaker's final formulation.

Speaker #1:

1. and um you need to serve when you serve, you need to serve behind the line, not over it.

2. and then um in order to um in order to score over there you in or ok when you serve and it goes over the net, and if the other players do not hit it or if they can't get it and it's in the in the lines, then it's a point.

Speaker #2:

1. but usually the stadiums cost maybe thirty or a lot of dollars a lot of millions of dollars to put into it.

2. and they can play in any kind of weather even except for snow because they don't play in the snow.

3. and a baseball game should last a major league baseball game should last three hours.

Speaker #3:

1. and and then there's I don't know how many people play in pro.

2. but I we usually play five on five like at school like in sports for school.

3. and um that's about it.

Speaker #4:

1. and he asks Peter if he would if Mike to switch jobs with him because his sh uh shoulder was sore.

2. and he was like, "No, I don't wanna lose take a chance on losing my turn on the grill."

3. he could say, "Okay but I get but one when one time when it's your time turn to be on the grill, you you need to let me you cannot have a turn to use the grill when it's your turn, but this time I will do your garbage for you if you let me have it when you take your turn to use the grill."

Speaker #5:

1. he could say, "Bob um you know you were supposed to help us with this project and when you don't participate in the group, it frustrates me because it makes our group look bad and I'd appreciate it if you'd participate in the group."

2. um he unless Bob's an absolutely nasty person, he should get some kind of good results because he was pretty polite about it and yeah.

Exercise 13–3. Calculating Clausal Density (CD)

Solve the following problems using the information that is provided.

1. 45 main clauses; 24 subordinate clauses; 45 C-units.   CD = _____

2. 82 main clauses; 68 subordinate clauses; 82 C-units.   CD = _____

3. 14 relative clauses; 20 adverbial clauses; 9 nominal clauses; 47 main clauses; 42 C-units.   CD = _____

4. 0 relative clauses; 17 adverbial clauses; 14 nominal clauses; 35 main clauses; 25 C-units.   CD = _____

5. 15 relative clauses; 25 adverbial clauses; 16 nominal clauses; 60 main clauses; 60 C-units.   CD = _____

6. 10 adverbial clauses; 6 relative clauses; 9 nominal clauses; 4 infinitive clauses; 5 gerund clauses; 5 participial clauses; 24 main clauses; 24 C-units.   CD = _____

7. 9 adverbial clauses; 0 relative clauses; 4 nominal clauses; 2 infinitive clauses; 0 gerund clauses; 0 participial clauses; 16 main clauses; 16 C-units.   CD = _____

8. 4 adverbial clauses; 2 relative clauses; 2 nominal clauses; 4 infinitive clauses; 0 gerund clauses; 0 participial clauses; 12 main clauses; 12 C-units.   CD = _____

CHAPTER 14

Analyzing Language Samples from Adolescents

Below are language samples (from the author's files) that were elicited from adolescents with typical language development. To elicit the samples, tasks were used that were described in Chapter 5 of this book. For each sample, indicate the types of main and subordinate clauses that occur, using the following codes: MC, ADV, REL, NOM, INF, PRT, GER.

E = examiner; C = adolescent

SAMPLE #1: CONVERSATION

Boy, Age 14 Years

MLCU = 9.93   CD = 1.70

E What would you like to tell me about yourself?

E For example, what could you tell me about school, or your family or friends or pets?

C (Um) at school I try [_____] to stay [_____] inclined.

C But I kind of get [_____] bored because I find [_____] it somewhat boring.

C At home I try [_____] to do [_____] my chores.

C But I don't [_____] because (I don't really need any) I don't have
    [_____] anything to do [_____] with the money after I get [_____] it.

C And (um) I hang [_____] out with (a) a pretty tight group of friends.

E Are they all in cross-country?

C (Um) one of them is [_____].

C And one of them is thinking [_____] about it.

C But they haven't really decided [_____] yet.

E How long have you been in cross-country?

C (Um) sixth grade.

E So two years.

E This is your second year?

C (Yes) no, this is [_____] my third.

C Started [_____] in sixth.

E Okay.

E And do you like it?

C (Um) It's [_____] a nice warm-up for track, which I'm [_____] more
    into 'cause I'm [_____] (kind of) better at track.

E Okay.

E What's your favorite track event?

C (Um) Pole vault.

E No way!

E Isn't that when you launch yourself over a tall pole?

C Yeah.

E You do that?

C (nods).

E Wow.

E Do you go to competitions for it?

C (Um) Well you're not allowed [_____] to do [_____] pole vault as a track event at other middle schools because I think [_____] McArthur (is the only) has [_____] the only (pole vault for like a) pole vault coach for middle school.

E So you can't compete with anyone.

C No.

E But you have a head start on competing.

C Yeah, I have [_____] a really big head start since I'm [_____] (like) the best person in my grade right now.

C There's [_____] not really a lot of other people who do [_____] it, just two of my friends.

E What do you have to know to do pole vault well?

C (Um) You have [_____] to have [_____] good timing.

C (Uh) You have [_____] to be [_____] able to relax [_____] because if you (like) tighten [_____] your abs when you're trying [_____] to turn [_____] upside down to go [_____] over the pole, you'll [_____] end up pulling [_____] on the bar and you might stretch [_____] a muscle in your shoulder, which hurts [_____].

C I've done [_____] that.

E You have?

E You stretched the muscle in your shoulder in pole vault?

C Yeah.

E Have you had any other track injuries?

C (Um well like) Yes, most of them are [_____] just (like) twisting [_____] ankles in long jump and stuff, though.

C They don't hurt [_____] as bad.

C It really hurts [_____].

E How long does a twisted ankle take to recover?

C Like a day or two.

E Oh cool.

E But then you're back running full speed?

C I actually normally run [_____] with a twisted ankle.

C It kind of helps [_____] stretch [_____] it out I think [_____].

C But I try [_____] not to put [_____] a whole bunch of weight on it.

E That's really cool.

SAMPLE #2: CONVERSATION

Girl, Age 14 Years

MLCU = 9.41   CD = 1.59

E I am going to ask you a little bit about yourself.

C Well, I wish [_____] I worked [_____].

C But I don't [_____].

C I have been trying [_____] to find [_____] a job this summer.

C But it appears [_____] no one is hiring [_____] (um) inexperienced 14-year-olds.

C (Um) I baby sit [_____] for a kid named [_____] Jacob.

C And he's [_____] really nice.

C He's [_____] ten and pretty mature.

C So it's [_____] kind of like being [_____] paid [_____] (like) six dollars an hour to (um) play [_____] video games and watch [_____] TV with him and stuff.

C (Um my school) My school is [_____] Westminster_Middle_School.

C (Um it's uh) It's [_____] an okay school.

C I think [_____] that it's [_____] a better fit for me than Southampton (but um it's).

E Why do you think that?

C (Uh) Well (we just) because (um) I was made [_____] fun of a lot when I was [_____] in fifth and sixth grades.

C So at Southampton (I would have had) I feel [_____] like there is [_____] just a more unfriendly atmosphere there.

C I'm [_____] not sure that I really like [_____] the friends I have [_____] at my school (um).

C But I'm going [_____] into Woodbury_High_School.

C And (um) that's going [_____] to be [_____] a new experience for me (you know).

C Because I've never been [_____] to high school before.

C (Um) Actually, I'm [_____] quite familiar with one part of Woodbury_High_School.

C (I um) I am [_____] a theatre person.

C So (like um) I've been [_____] in a summer camp where they basically use [_____] the entire (like) theatre and choir wing of Woodbury_High_School.

C And (I've been up) I've performed [_____] on that stage at least three times.

C (Um) I'm [_____] really into theatre and acting and stuff.

C In fact, (I was) my (uh) first professional role was [_____] in Sleeping_Beauty.

C (Um) It's [_____] the only professional role I've had [_____] yet because there's [_____] just nothing up for kids although I am auditioning [_____] for My_Fair_Lady.

C (Um uh) So we'll see [_____] how that goes [_____].

C (But um) I was [_____] in Sleeping_Beauty as a fairy.

C And (uh) over a hundred kids tried [_____] out.

C So I was [_____] pretty unprofessional.

C So I'm [_____] not quite sure how I got [_____] in.

C But (uh) it was [_____] pretty fun.

C But so yeah.

C I performed [_____] on the community_center stage (um).

E When was that?

C That was [_____] when I was [_____] in fifth grade.

C I think [_____] I was going [_____] into fifth grade.

C Yeah, I was going [_____] into fifth grade.

C And (um) I was [_____] just a fairy (but).

E And did you speak?

C (Um) I sang [_____] on stage.

C But I didn't have [_____] any solos or anything.

C (Yeah I was) Yeah (uh) I ate [_____] like a mountain load of candy before every performance, which was [_____] not good for my voice I'm [_____] sure (still but).

SAMPLE #3: CONVERSATION

Boy, Age 14 Years

MLCU = 7.76   CD = 1.18

E What would you like to tell me about yourself?

E For example, what could you tell me about school, or your family or friends or pets?

C (Well I have) My family is [_____] really close to me.

C Like (um) all my cousins and uncles and aunts live [_____] in Roseburg with me.

C And I see [_____] most of them almost every day.

C (Um).

E How many do you have?

C (I have) Both my grandma and grandpas live [_____] in Roseburg.

C I have [_____] I think [_____] three aunts that live [_____] here and two uncles maybe.

E Do any of your aunts and uncles live elsewhere?

C (Uh) Yeah, actually I have [_____] an aunt and uncle in Bend.

C But I see [_____] them like five or six times a year.

E So you have a lot of cousins?

C Yeah, I have [_____] a lot of cousins.

E That sounds fun to me.

C (Um) Well (like) most of my family is [_____] (like) teachers or doctors.

C And then (my) one of my uncles that lives [_____] in Bend is [_____] an engineer.

E Oh cool.

C (Um) What else.

E Do you have pets?

C (Yeah I have) My sister has [_____] a turtle.

C And I have [_____] a dog.

E A turtle and a dog!

E Does the dog get along with the turtle?

C Well I guess [_____].

C He doesn't try [_____] to bite [_____] him or anything.

E That's good.

E At least the turtle will be able to crawl into its shell.

E Does it live in a cage?

C Yeah, but (he like) sometimes my sister will let [_____] him out in the
    back yard to walk [_____] around in the summer.

E Is it big?

C Yeah, (it's like) well when we got [_____] it, it was [_____] like that
    small.

C But now it's [_____] like that big.

E It's amazing how they grow!

C And it's [_____] supposed to be [_____] (like) like four feet by four feet
    when it gets [_____] older.

C And they live [_____] like one hundred years.

E No way!

E How old is it now?

C (Um) Like three?

E Wow!

E It seems like it has grown a lot in three years.

C Uhhuh, yeah.

E So it will be really big, like one of those Galapagos Islands turtles.

E And so what is your dog like?

E What do you like to do with your dog?

C Well my dog is [_____] very small.

C He's [_____] a Chihuahua.

C He isn't [_____] really active.

C He just sits [_____] around all day.

E Is it a puppy or is it older?

C Well it's [_____] like six I think [_____] now.

C But he is [_____] I think [_____] a teacup Chihuahua.

C I'm [_____] not sure.

E Really!

E What's your favorite thing about him?

C (Um) I don't know [_____].

C Probably how (like) one second he can be [_____] like totally calm.

C But the other he will be [_____] very playful.

E He's unpredictable?

C And he listens [_____] pretty well.

E That's nice.

SAMPLE #4: MICE IN COUNCIL NARRATIVE RETELL

Boy, Age 14 Years

MLCU = 9.12   CD = 1.88

E Can you retell the story?

C (Uh) I could try [_____], yes.

C So (uh) these mice are living [_____] in fear of the cat.

C That('s uh) happens [_____] a lot (I guess).

C And so (um) they decided [_____] to make [_____] a council because of the name of the story to try [_____] and figure [_____] out a way to (uh) solve [_____] this problem.

C Because (you know) they're losing [_____] a lot of people getting eaten [_____] up by the cat.

C So they keep [_____] talking [_____] and talking [_____].

C And nothing seems [_____] to work [_____] (to work that would work).

C And one (mice) mouse was [_____] (uh) smart (I guess).

C (To uh) mice decided [_____] to (uh) make [_____] it so that the cat could be heard [_____] by putting [_____] a bell around his neck.

C They thought [_____] it was [_____] an amazing idea.

C So they applauded [_____].

C And he gave [_____] a couple bows.

C And then (uh the) it was passed [_____] that they would do [_____] this.

C 'Cause they have [_____] a little council.

C But (uh) then one old mouse that's [_____] wise (uh, uh) was (uh) congratulating [_____] him and thought [_____] of a question.

C (Uh) who would put [_____] the bell around the (mouse or) cat.

C And (uh) that's [_____] a good question.

E Awesome, nicely retold.

SAMPLE #5: MICE IN COUNCIL NARRATIVE RETELL

Girl, Age 14 Years
MLCU = 12.13   CD = 2.53

C (So) the mice were [_____] always in fear of this cat because (they'd always) he'd always approach [_____] them and try [_____] and eat [_____] them.

C And he'd toy [_____] with them and torture [_____] them.

C So the mice called [_____] together a council meeting.

C And they discussed [_____] many plans.

C But none of them seemed [_____] (to work or) like they were going [_____] to work [_____].

C And then a very small young mouse (um) approached [_____] and said [_____] that his idea was [_____] to put [_____] a bell around the cat's neck so that whenever the cat came [_____] they would hear [_____] the bell tinkle [_____] and then they would know [_____] he was coming [_____] so they could escape [_____].

C And everyone thought [_____] it was [_____] a really great idea.

C And so (um) they applauded [_____] him.

C And he took [_____] a few bows.

C And then (um) a wise older mouse stood [_____] up.

C And (said) this is [_____] basically what he said [_____].

C This is [_____] truly a great plan.

C And (um) only a genius could figure [_____] out a plan so simple (that we could) that we would have overlooked [_____].

C And he says [_____] so now the question is [_____] who's going [_____] to put [_____] the bell on the cat.

C So basically things are [_____] easier said [_____] than done [_____].

SAMPLE #6: MONKEY AND DOLPHIN NARRATIVE RETELL

Boy, Age 14 Years

MLCU = 9.74   CD = 1.84

E Can you tell that story back to me?

C (Uh) so (uh) I guess [_____] it was [_____] a custom to bring [_____] monkeys and other creatures along with them to amuse [_____] the (sailor) sailors.

C So one guy brought [_____] a monkey onto his boat.

C And they were sailing [_____] around somewhere (Uh) by (Greek) Greece (I guess).

C And (uh) there was [_____] a storm.

C The ship crashed [_____].

C And everyone was [_____] in the water.

C And they were swimming [_____] towards shore.

C And so was [_____] the monkey.

C And then a dolphin, who must have [_____] bad eyesight to mistake [_____] a monkey for a man, (uh) swam [_____] up and grabbed [_____] the monkey with his back.

C And so the monkey had gotten [_____] onto him.

C And they're swimming [_____] there.

C And he asked [_____] him if he was [_____] (a uh citizen) a
   Athenian.

C And the monkey said [_____] 'yes' (you know) trying [_____] to trick
   [_____] this dolphin because he's trying [_____] to live [_____] on.

C And the dolphin asked [_____] him if he knew [_____] something or
   someone.

C And the monkey, (you know) thinking [_____] that oh yeah this must
   be [_____] (uh) someone.

C Like oh yeah I know [_____] him.

C He's [_____] a dear friend.

C And the dolphin knew [_____] that he was lying [_____].

C So instead of saving [_____] him, he plunged [_____] down to the
   bottom to leave [_____] the monkey to his fate.

E Very nice.

SAMPLE #7: MONKEY AND DOLPHIN NARRATIVE RETELL

Girl, Age 14 Years

MLCU = 13.29   CD = 2.21

C (Um) so it used [_____] to be [_____] (um) a custom that sailors would
   take [_____] on with them animals like a monkey or a dog to keep
   [_____] them entertained [_____] on their long voyage.

C So on one particular (um) voyage, they took [_____] with them a
   monkey.

C And when they were [_____] off the coast of Sunium, there was
   [_____] a terrible shipwreck.

C And everyone was turned [_____] overboard, including [_____] the
   monkey.

C So a nearby dolphin (mis) mistook [_____] the monkey for a man.

C And so he came [_____] to his rescue.

C And then the dolphin asked [_____] him if he knew [_____] Piraeus, which was [_____] also the name of the harbor off of Athens.

C And (um) he said [_____] yes I'm [_____] (a) an Athenian.

C I'm [_____] from one of the first families that was [_____] here.

C And he said [_____] yes I knew [_____] Piraeus.

C He's [_____] one of my oldest friends.

C And the dolphin knew [_____] then that he was (uh) not telling [_____] the truth, that he was lying [_____].

C And so he dove [_____] deep into the water and left [_____] the monkey to his fate.

C And so the moral of the story would be [_____] people who pretend [_____] (uh) to be [_____] someone else basically end [_____] up in deep water.

SAMPLE #8: WHAT HAPPENED ONE DAY, NARRATIVE ESSAY

Boy, Age 17 Years

MLTU = 13.68   CD = 2.58

C One day a long time ago, my friend Jack and I went [_____] on a camping trip all by ourselves.

C We set [_____] up camp and went fishing [_____] to try [_____] and catch [_____] our dinner.

C I caught [_____] two fish while Jack caught [_____] three.

C We were getting [_____] ready to leave [_____] when I looked [_____] up the river and saw [_____] this big dark blurry figure run [_____] off into the bushes.

C I didn't think [_____] anything of it.

C I just thought [_____] it was [_____] an elk.

C On our way back to the camp, Jack started [_____] taunting [_____] me and bragging [_____] about how he was [_____] a better fisherman than I was [_____] because he caught [_____] three fish while I only caught [_____] two.

C We got [_____] back to camp.

C And I started [_____] a fire to cook [_____] the fish.

C I always started [_____] the fires.

C I was [_____] the best fire starter.

C We cooked [_____] some of our fish and put [_____] the rest in the ice chest for breakfast.

C We made [_____] our beds and went [_____] to sleep [_____].

C Jack was still bragging [_____] about his fish.

C When I woke [_____] in the morning, I opened [_____] my eyes to see [_____] Bigfoot eating [_____] our fish.

C As I leaned [_____] over to wake [_____] up Jack, it looked [_____] at me and ran [_____] off into the forest.

C Just like that, our camping trip turned [_____] into a hunt for rock solid proof of Bigfoot.

C After three days trying [_____] and failing [_____] to find [_____] Bigfoot anywhere, we gave [_____] up and went [_____] home.

C Ever since that day, I always have been [_____] sure to bring [_____] three things camping with me, a gun, a camera, and a better type of fishing bait.

SAMPLE #9: FAVORITE GAME OR SPORT EXPOSITORY TASK

Boy, Age 13 Years

MLTU = 10.16   CD = 1.67

E What is your favorite game or sport?

C My favorite sport in school would be [_____] wrestling.

E Why is wrestling your favorite sport?

C Well the (uh) coaches are [_____] really nice and everything.

C (we got got uh) We started [_____] out doing [_____] these (like uh) extra things.

C And (then uh and) then eventually I did [_____] everything and got [_____] good at it.

C So started [_____] getting [_____] gold medals and stuff.

E I'm not too familiar with the sport of wrestling, so I would like you to tell me all about it.

E For example, tell me what the goals are, and how many people may play a match.

E Also, tell me about the rules that players need to follow.

E Tell me everything you can think of about the sport of wrestling so that someone who has never played before would know how to play.

C (we) You start [_____] on a mat.

C You warm up [_____].

C You go [_____] over to the mat.

C You shake [_____] hands.

C And the ref blows [_____] the whistle.

C And when you wrestle [_____], you start [_____] out neutral.

C And (you have to um you have to) you take [_____] the guy down by getting [_____] control of him while their hands or their feet are [_____] on the mat.

C And if you're taking [_____] a guy down (you can't like if you come around the back), you can't just pick [_____] them up and slap [_____] them on the mat.

C Otherwise it's [_____] unnecessary roughness.

C you get docked [_____] off a point.

C and if they are [_____] (uh) too injured to wrestle [_____] then they win [_____] the match.

C and (um) it's [_____] really big on sportsmanship.

C so you can't go [_____] over and yell [_____] at the ref or yell [_____] at (the) them.

C Otherwise you'll get kicked [_____] for the next tournament.

C and (um yeah you also you have um you have to) you have [_____] to shake [_____] hands because it's [_____] pretty much sportsmanship to do [_____] that.

C and once you get [_____] the take down on them, you (um) try [_____] to break [_____] them down to their back.

C and you get [_____] them past a 45 degree angle.

C and you get [_____] near full points.

C then (uh) for 3 points, it's [_____] like 2 points.

C and (uh 5 points/s it/'s like 3 poin er uh) 5 seconds it's [_____] 3 points.

C and then after that, (you uh for how long) you hold [_____] them down.

C and it's [_____] about a 2 second pin.

C and if you get [_____] both their shoulders down and (uh them you uh) if you pin [_____] them, you get [_____] to shake [_____] hands.

C and you win [_____].

C but there's [_____] also points.

C like for college, there's [_____] advantage time which is [_____] where (like somebody if) somebody was riding [_____] a person for a long time.

C and they get [_____] points.

C (but once they go neutral then the timing down and stuff).

C (so uh they have to kinda like) that's [_____] how it goes [_____] with the advantage time.

C They get [_____] certain amount of points at the end for advantage time and stuff.

C (uh) it's [_____] pretty much big on sportsmanship.

C and it's [_____] pretty easy to learn [_____].

C also you can't lock [_____] hands while they're [_____] down around their waist (but) like around the leg (or around the ar).

C but around the arm is [_____] okay.

C (and stuff like that and can't like uh) in freestyle you can do [_____] that because it's [_____] a big part of freestyle.

E Now I would like you to tell me what a player should do in order to win the sport of wrestling.

E In other words, what are some key strategies that every good player should know?

C you just try [_____] to turn [_____] them so you get [_____] back points.

C and (uh once second) once both their shoulders touch [_____] the mat, they're [_____] pinned.

E Do they have to go all the way down?

C no you just have [_____] to get [_____] their shoulders to touch [_____].

E How long is a match?

C (um match/s are usually like in reg) I think [_____] they're [_____] the same in everyone.

C so (they) for middle school, it's [_____] (like) about (like uh) three minutes or maybe four minutes or something like that.

C for high school it's [_____] six minutes.

C and college I'm [_____] not sure.

C I think [_____] it's [_____] about the same as high school or (like) 30 seconds more or something.

E So a match isn't all that long.

C yeah it's [_____] not too hard (it's just) if you're [_____] conditioned well and you have [_____] a good work ethic.

C then you'll probably do [_____] well in wrestling.

C but if you don't try [_____] your hardest, you're never going [_____] to get [_____] anywhere.

C yeah it's [_____] pretty much you can beat [_____] guys that are [_____] strong as long as you have [_____] a good technique.

C (but strength is kinda like) some people can just do [_____] bad technique and just knock [_____] you down and (um) then pin [_____] me and stuff.

C but most of the time you can get [_____] them.

E What about freestyle?

C (well in freestyle it's just you) I don't know [_____] much about freestyle.

C but you just touch [_____] (their both) their shoulders on the mat.

C and you win [_____].

C or you win [_____] by points at the end of the match.

C (same with collegiate except in collegiate it like 2 points pin).

C and (then like you'll uh and) if you don't pin [_____] through the whole match, then you win [_____] by a certain amount of points.

C and then you get [_____] a certain amount of points for your team.

C but you can also technical [_____] them which is [_____] (like) when (you uh if) you (get) gain [_____] (like) 15 points more than them.

C then they stop [_____] the match.

C and you win [_____].

SAMPLE #10: PEER CONFLICT RESOLUTION
SCIENCE FAIR TASK

Girl, Age 17 Years

MLCU = 15.40   CD = 3.40

E Now I'd like you to tell the story back to me, in your own words.

E Try to tell me everything you can remember about the story.

C The teacher gave [_____] the four girls an assignment to work [_____] together on a science project.

C And they decided [_____] they were going [_____] to make [_____] a model airplane that could actually fly [_____].

C And everyone worked [_____] on it except for one girl named [_____] Melanie.

C And (it made Debbie angry or um) it made [_____] her indifferent because she wouldn't do [_____] the work.

E What is the main problem here?

C (um) not everyone was participating [_____] equally or helping [_____] participating [_____].

E Why is that a problem?

C Well if one person doesn't do [_____] anything and they're [_____] still in the group, they're still going [_____] to get [_____] the same grade.

C Or they're still going [_____] to be [_____] in that group as all the people that worked [_____] as hard.

C But they didn't contribute [_____] to it at all.

C So the other people may feel [_____] like they didn't deserve [_____] it.

E What is a good way for Debbie to deal with Melanie?

C (um) I guess [_____] Debbie could ask [_____] Melanie why she didn't want [_____] to help [_____] or maybe she wanted [_____] to do [_____] something different than what they wanted [_____] to do [_____].

C Maybe that's [_____] the reason she didn't want [_____] to help [_____].

C (or) And if that didn't work [_____], then she could ask [_____] the teacher to help [_____] them.

E Why is that a good way for Debbie to deal with Melanie?

C Because it's [_____] calm.

C She's not going [_____] to be [_____] like yelling [_____] at her.

C They're going [_____] to try [_____] to compromise [_____] about it so that the three girls can do [_____] what they want [_____] to do [_____].

C But Melanie can also help [_____] since they're all contributing [_____] to it.

E What do you think will happen if Debbie does that?

C (um) Maybe Melanie will say [_____] that she didn't want [_____] to make [_____] an airplane or (she um) she wanted [_____] to do [_____] something different.

C And so maybe they could interact [_____] that way and find [_____] out what the problem was [_____] so Melanie could help [_____] do [_____] something.

E How do you think they both will feel if Debbie does that?

C I think [_____] that they would kind of feel [_____] more relaxed and not so uptight about her not helping [_____] or maybe Melanie not getting [_____] to do [_____] what she wants [_____] to do [_____].

C Maybe they would both feel [_____] more comfortable about the problem or talking [_____] about it.

SAMPLE #11: PEER CONFLICT RESOLUTION
FAST FOOD RESTAURANT TASK

Girl, Age 17 Years

MLCU = 11.63   CD = 2.21

E Now I'd like you to tell the story back to me, in your own words.

C (um Jane and Kathy) Jane is going [_____] to cook [_____] the food on the grill.

C And Kathy is going [_____] to take [_____] out the garbage.

C But her arm really hurts [_____].

C And she wants [_____] to switch [_____] jobs.

C But Jane doesn't want [_____] to lose [_____] her spot at the grill.

E What is the main problem here?

C The main problem is [_____] that (maybe) maybe Jane doesn't want
   [_____] to give [_____] up her spot.

C Maybe they could just switch [_____] for a minute for her to take
   [_____] out the garbage.

C Or maybe she could help [_____] Kathy take [_____] out the garbage.

C The main problem is [_____] that (they don't want to) Jane doesn't
   want [_____] to switch [_____] jobs.

C But maybe she can just help [_____] Kathy instead do [_____] the grill.

E Why is that a problem?

C Because she said [_____] that she didn't want [_____] to give [_____]
   up her spot at the grill.

C So obviously she didn't want [_____] to give [_____] up her spot at
   the grill.

C And (maybe) I don't know [_____] why.

E What is a good way for Jane to deal with Kathy?

C Well Jane could help [_____] Kathy take [_____] the garbage out.

C Or someone else could do [_____] it.

E Why is that a good way for Jane to deal with Kathy?

C Because they could both get [_____] their jobs done and help [_____]
   each other.

E What do you think will happen if Jane does that?

C I think [_____] that Kathy would really appreciate [_____] it if Jane
   helped [_____] her (and) and maybe in turn Kathy would help [_____]
   Jane if she wanted [_____] it.

C (or um) Then they could both get [_____] their jobs done.

E How do you think they both will feel if Jane does that?

C They'll both feel [_____] (like) happy that everything got done [_____] or happy (that they solved) that they could help [_____] each other and solve [_____] the problems.

SAMPLE #12: NATURE OF FRIENDSHIP EXPOSITORY ESSAY

Girl, Age 17 Years

MLTU = 12.48   CD = 2.28

C To me, friendship is [_____] a relationship between two or more people that like [_____] spending [_____] time with each other.

C A friend is [_____] someone you can talk [_____] to when there is [_____] no other.

C You can tell [_____] them your secrets.

C And they will always have [_____] your back.

C If the world didn't have [_____] friendship, then relationships and social status wouldn't mean [_____] a thing.

C The world would be [_____] full of people that don't like [_____] each other.

C And most of all, there wouldn't be [_____] anyone to talk [_____] with.

C Friends mostly keep [_____] you occupied.

C If I didn't have [_____] friends, then my life would lack [_____] the excitement everyone needs [_____].

C I would just wake [_____] up, go [_____] to school, come home [_____] and either watch [_____] TV or do [_____] nothing.

C With friends, it's [_____] like our lives are [_____] all intertwined.

C And if one of us is doing [_____] something exciting, then the rest should be [_____] in on it as well.

C Living [_____] a boring life isn't [_____] worth it.

C Usually friends share [_____] common interests.

C Either it being [_____] culture, neighborhood, or personalities, they are [_____] usually like the other.

C Friendship to children is [_____] having [_____] someone to play [_____] with.

C Usually it's [_____] a person from school or a neighbor.

C For teenagers like me, friendship means [_____] someone to talk [_____] to when we get [_____] in a fight with our parents, boyfriend, or girlfriends.

C Adults see [_____] friendship as more of a companionship.

C If they have [_____] common interest in things, then they are [_____] more than likely to become [_____] friends.

C Or they have just been [_____] friends for a really long time.

C Usually people are [_____] friends one year then just are [_____] n't the next.

C People grow [_____] up and change [_____] and make [_____] new friends everyday.

C Sometimes friends just drift [_____] apart over the years.

C Other times, friends can do [_____] or say [_____] something that doesn't make [_____] them trustworthy.

C The usual result is [_____] a misunderstanding or someone gets [_____] hurt.

C The best of friends are [_____] the ones that stay [_____] in touch for a really long time.

C There have been [_____] cases of people being [_____] friends since they were [_____] three, and now at age sixty they are [_____] still together.

C Friendships come [_____] and go [_____], and depending [_____] on what kind of friendship it is [_____], can last [_____] a lifetime.

SAMPLE #13: CIRCUS CONTROVERSY PERSUASIVE ESSAY

Boy, Age 17 Years

MLTU = 15.43   CD = 3.00

C Should animals perform [_____] in circuses?

C I believe [_____] that being [_____] trained to do [_____] tricks and to entertain [_____] audiences is [_____] a very good use for animals.

C There are [_____], however, a couple of sides on this subject.

C Some people think [_____] only of the entertainment with no concern for the animals' needs.

C Circuses may not feed [_____] the animals well or give [_____] them adequate space to live [_____] just for a little extra profit.

C It's [_____] also possible that they use [_____] dangerous training techniques.

C These are [_____] all negative aspects on animals performing [_____] in circuses.

C There is [_____] also a good side to having [_____] circus animals.

C They can provide [_____] much entertainment for both adults and children, performing [_____] stunts, tricks, and acrobatics, jumping [_____] through fiery hoops, walking [_____] on hind legs, things you don't usually see [_____] your pets doing [_____].

C This can also help [_____] to eliminate [_____] any fears children might have [_____] of the performing animals.

C Looking [_____] back at this reasoning and the impressions it gives [_____] us, I can see [_____] that there is [_____] an easy solution to get [_____] rid of the negative aspects.

C Allow [_____] for the animals to perform [_____] in circuses, but only if they are [_____] treated well, given [_____] enough food, large enough living areas, and trained [_____] without using [_____] too harsh punishment.

C Using [_____] this method, there are [_____] only positive reasons.

C So why not have [_____] animals perform [_____] in circuses?

SAMPLE #14: CIRCUS CONTROVERSY PERSUASIVE ESSAY

Girl, Age 18 Years

MLTU = 11.69   CD = 2.38

C I feel [_____] that animals performing [_____] for our entertainment is [_____] a bad idea!

C We have [_____] many other forms of entertainment in this day and age.

C We do not need [_____] to force [_____] wild animals to do [_____] things for our entertainment.

C The animals that are [_____] part of circuses do not have [_____] the proper habitat that they need [_____].

C They do not have [_____] space that they need [_____].

C And they have been known [_____] to become [_____] violent.

C I do not have [_____] a problem with people performing [_____], with cats and dogs, even horses.

C But all of these are [_____] domestic animals.

C Tigers, bears, and elephants should not be [_____] locked [_____] in small cages, forced [_____] to do [_____] tricks, and be [_____] poorly treated [_____].

C There is [_____] no reason that people and domestic animals could not give [_____] just as good of a performance.

C Wild animals are [_____] just that, wild.

C They need [_____] to be [_____] in habitats that are [_____] suitable for them.

C They need [_____] to be [_____] fed [_____] right and let [_____] to use [_____] their instincts.

C Malnutrition, small confined areas, and entertainment for people is [_____] not what these creatures are [_____] on this earth for.

C They are [_____] animals, not actors.

C And we need [_____] to remember [_____] this.

APPENDIX A

Answer Keys for Chapter Exercises

ANSWERS FOR CHAPTER 10:
TYPES OF WORDS AND PHRASES

Exercise 10–1. Identifying Words in Passages

In passages 1–6, circle all of the *nouns* including *gerunds* and *proper nouns* (but not pronouns).

1. **Computers** can do **lots** of **things**. They can add **millions** of **numbers** in the **twinkling** of an **eye**. They can outwit chess **grandmasters**. They can guide **weapons** to their **targets**. They can book you onto a **plane** between a guitar-strumming **nun** and a nonsmoking physics **professor**. Some can even play the **bongos**. That's quite a **variety**! So if we're going to talk about **computers**, we'd better decide right now which of them we're going to look at, and how (Feynman, 1996, p. 1).

2. Most of the **luxuries**, and many of the so-called **comforts** of **life**, are not only not indispensable, but positive **hindrances** to the **elevation** of **mankind**. With **respect** to **luxuries** and **comforts**, the **wisest**

have ever lived a more simple and meager **life** than the **poor**. The ancient **philosophers**, Chinese, Hindoo, Persian, and Greek, were a **class** than which none has been poorer in outward **riches**, none so rich in inward (Thoreau, 2004, p. 14)

3. For a French **parent, education** is everything. The **child** must have as many and as important **certificates** of academic **attainment** as possible. In American and British business **life, experience** counts. In French **life**, the right **education** and the right **certificates** count. This is why some experienced American and British **teachers** wishing to work in **France** are horrified to find their **experience** downgraded because they do not have the equivalent degree **certificate** to the French one (Tomalin, 2003, p. 93).

4. There are two **kinds** of **knowledge**. One is the everyday **kind** of **knowledge** we have of the **world**, which we get through our **senses** (usually called "empirical" **knowledge**). **Plato** thought that this **kind** of **knowledge** was useful enough for ordinary **people** to go about their everyday **lives**. But it wasn't the real **thing**. Like **Heraclitus, Pythagoras**, and maybe **Socrates, Plato** thought that the empirical **world** was a **kind** of **illusion**, a **veil** that hid the real **truth** from us (Robinson & Groves, 2005, p. 62).

5. **Plato** was probably the greatest **philosopher** of all **time**, and the first to collect all **sorts** of different **ideas** and **arguments** into **books** that everyone can read. He wanted to know about everything and constantly pestered his fellow **philosophers** for **answers** to his disturbing **questions**. He also had resolute **ideas** of his own, some of which seem sensible enough, and some of which now seem extremely odd. But, from the **start**, he knew that "**doing philosophy**" was a very special **activity** (Robinson & Groves, 2005, p. 3).

6. I propose that **educationalists** should no longer conceive of **children** as passive, empty jam **jars** who need to be stuffed with

information, but as independently-minded problem **solvers** who need to be continually challenged (John Dewey; Robinson & Groves, 2004, p. 111).

In passages 7–12, circle all of the *adjectives* including the *participles*:

7. The legacy of **Scotland's tumultuous** and often **violent** history can be found in its **extraordinary** array of **prehistoric** sites, **religious** ruins, and other **historic** attractions. Today these relics offer visitors **intriguing** insights into **some** of the **defining** battles, heroes, and **forgotten** worlds of the country's **rich** and **turbulent** past (Wilson & Murphy, 2008, p. 274).

8. Once Oregon was thought to be **immune** to earthquakes. Today we know that we have them in **three different** flavors—**devastating subduction** earthquakes like the **1700** catastrophe, **deep intraplate** earthquakes like the **Puget Sound** temblors of 1949 and 2001, and **sharp local** jolts like the **Spring Break** Quake of 1993 (Sullivan, 2008, p. 67).

9. **Some** artists are **finite** draftsmen with **meticulous drawing** skills. **Other** artists are storytellers. A few invent a **new** lens of perception. But Sarkis Antikajian is a painter. His work is a **bodacious** celebration of brush **dipped** in paint and **spread** across canvas. While **some** painters claim they paint light, Sarkis Antikajian paints energy. He leaves his viewer **breathless** by the onslaught on his transcription. His **masterful** use of **intense** chroma ravishes the **visual** cortex in a **heady** embrace. Sarkis wields color with the **same** bravado **employed** by the trumpeter Maynard Ferguson when he plays C above **high** C (Moffet, 2006, pp. 18–19).

10. The **ancient** Greeks made **extensive** use of honey in salves and potions, in **prepared** dishes, to make perfume, as libations for the dead, and to appease the gods. Bee-keepers numbered among their ranks the philosopher Aristotle; for Hippocrates, the father of

medicine, honey was a **favorite** remedy. The followers of Pythagoras lived on a diet of bread and honey—and seemed to far outlive any of their contemporaries (Style, 1993, p. 14).

11. **French** culture once dominated **Western** civilization. From about 1650 to about 1920, the **upper** classes in **several** countries preferred French to their own **native** languages. French was the **official** language for **diplomatic** negotiations and **much government** business. The achievements of **French** writers, artists, architects, and composers were widely admired and imitated. Since then, **other** cultures have moved to the forefront. English has overtaken French as the most widely **spoken** language (Harris, 1989, p. 167).

12. Mister Fox was just about **famished** and **thirsty** too, when he stole into a vineyard where the **sun-ripened** grapes were hanging upon a trellis in a **tempting** show, but too **high** for him to reach. He took a run and a jump, **snapping** at the **nearest** bunch, but missed. Again and again he jumped, only to miss the **luscious** prize. At last, **worn** out with his efforts, he retreated, **muttering**: "Well, I never really wanted those grapes anyway. I am **sure** they are **sour**, and perhaps **wormy** in the bargain" (Grosset & Dunlap, 1947, p. 14).

In passages 13–17, circle all of the *finite verbs*:

13. Trieste, set on a gulf with rolling hills as a backdrop, **is** the most important seaport on the northern Adriatic. Because of its geographic position and its history, the cooking of Trieste **is** eclectic. *Gnocchetti di fegato*, liver dumplings, **are** a reminder of Austrian ties. Venezia's influence **is** apparent in its many risotto, including its own version of *risi e bisi*. It also **has** its own variation of *brodetto*, the fish stew so popular along the entire Italian coastline. Made with local fish, the sauce **contains** vinegar, wine, and sometimes tomatoes, and **is** always **served** with grilled polenta. There **are** many rich desserts. Typical **are** *strucoli*, similar to strudel, which like *preniz*, an Easter

specialty, **are made** with a variety of ingredients (Luciano et al., 1991, p. 87).

14. When first I **took** up my abode in the woods, that **is, began** to spend my nights as well as days there, which, by accident, **was** on Independence Day, or the fourth of July, 1845, my house **was** not finished for winter, but **was** merely a defense against the rain, without plastering or chimney, the walls being of rough weather-stained boards, with wide chinks, which **made** it cool at night (Thoreau, 2004, p. 81).

15. The only house I **had been** the owner of before, if I **except** a boat, **was** a tent, which I **used** occasionally when making excursions in the summer, and this **is** still rolled up in my garret; but the boat, after passing from hand to hand, **has gone** down the stream of time. With this more substantial shelter about me, I **had made** some progress toward settling in the world (Thoreau, 2004, p. 82).

16. Sonja Kovalevsky (1850–1891), earlier known as Sophia Korvin-Krukovsky, **was** a gifted mathematician. She **was born** in Moscow to Russian nobility. She **left** Russia in 1868 because universities **were closed** to women. She **went** to Germany because she **wished** to study with Karl Weierstrass in Berlin. It **was said** that her early interest in mathematics **was** due in part to an odd wallpaper that **covered** her room in a summer house. Fascinated, she **spent** hours trying to make sense of it. The paper **turned** out to be lecture notes on higher mathematics purchased by her father during his student days (Smith, 1995, p. 479).

17. In his famous laboratory school at the University of Chicago, children **were** (and still **are**) **encouraged** to solve problems by inventing hypotheses and testing them. Dewey **thought** that art **should be encouraged** because it **stimulates** imaginative "solutions" to its own unique "problems" (Robinson & Groves, 2004, p. 111).

In passages 18–22, circle all of the *adverbs*.

18. Western Iran extends from the border with Armenia and Azerbaijan in the north to the industrial city of Ahvaz near the Gulf. **Culturally**, it is the **most** diverse part of Iran, with Azaris, Armenians, Loris, Bakhtiaris, and Kurds among the distinct ethnic groups you'll encounter. Despite this and a wealth of historical, religious, and cultural sights, stunning mountain scenery, and great trekking possibilities, few travelers see more than Tabriz. Pity them, then take advantage of the unspoilt expanses, and go yourself (Ham et al., 2006, p. 199).

19. The Middle East is home to some of the world's **most** significant cities—Jerusalem, Cairo, Damascus, Baghdad, and Istanbul. The ruins of the **once similarly** epic cities of history—Petra, Persepolis, Ephesus, Palmyra, Baalbek, Leptis Magna, and the bounty of ancient Egypt—also mark the passage of centuries in a region where the ancient world lives and breathes. The landscapes of the region are **equally** spellbinding, from the unrivalled seas of sand dunes and palm-fringed lakes in Libya's Sahara desert to the stunning mountains of the north, and the underwater world of the Red Sea (Ham et al., 2006, p. 4).

20. Mt. Fuji is the highest mountain in Japan and **by far** the **most** splendid, but during July and August (the open season) it is not a **dauntingly** hard climb. An athlete, it is said, could leave home in Tokyo in the morning, reach the peak and be home in time for dinner. Most people prefer to take it at a **more** leisurely pace, spending a night at the top and greeting the morning sun with a cry of "*Banzai!*" (Popham, 1992, p. 159).

21. I left the woods for as good a reason as I went there. **Perhaps** it seemed to me that I had **several** more lives to live, and could not spare **any** more time for that one. It is remarkable how **easily** and **insensibly** we fall into a particular route, and make a beaten

track for ourselves. I had not lived there a week before my feet wore a path from my door to the pond-side; and though it is five or six years since I trod it, it is **still quite** distinct. It is true, I fear that others may have fallen into it, and so helped to keep it open (Thoreau, 2004, p. 313).

22. John Dewey (1859–1952) was a systematic pragmatist or "instrumentalist" who believed that being "philosophical" **really** meant being **critically** intelligent and maintaining a "scientific" approach to human problems. Pragmatists like Dewey were great enthusiasts for the successes of science and its methods of inquiry. Dewey was convinced that philosophy could **also** play a key role in a creative American democracy by contributing to all kinds of knowledge in ethics, art, education, and the **newly** emerging social sciences. Like Pierce, Dewey was a theoretical "fallibilist," but **still firmly** a believer in the real possibility of practical progress in human affairs. Society can **only** progress if its members are educated to be intelligent and flexible (Robinson & Groves, 2004, p. 111).

In passage 23, circle all of the *prepositions*:

23. The year 1877 was an important one **in** the study **of** the planet Mars. The Red Planet came unusually close **to** Earth, affording astronomers an especially good view. **Of** particular note was the discovery, **by** U.S. Naval Observatory astronomer Asaph Hall, **of** the two moons circling Mars. But most exciting was the report **of** the Italian astronomer Giovanni Schiaparelli **on** his observations **of** a network **of** linear markings that he termed *canali*. **In** Italian, the word usually means "grooves" or "channels," but it can also mean "canals" (Chaisson & McMillan, 2005, p. 140).

In passages 24–25, circle all of the *pronouns*:

24. **This** country, with **its** institutions, belongs to the people **who** inhabit **it**. Whenever **they** shall grow weary of the existing

government, **they** can exercise **their** *constitutional* right of amending **it**, or **their** *revolutionary* right to dismember, or overthrow **it**. **I** cannot be ignorant of the fact **that** many worthy, and patriotic citizens are desirous of having the constitution amended (Emerson, 2009/1841, *Self-Reliance*, p. 41).

25. **All** the barnyard knew **that** the hen was indisposed. So **one** day, the cat decided to pay **her** a visit of condolence. Creeping up to **her** nest, the cat in **his** most sympathetic voice said, "How are **you**, **my** dear friend? **I** was so sorry to hear of **your** illness. Isn't **there** **something that I** can bring **you** to cheer **you** up and to help **you** feel like **yourself** again?" "Thank **you**," said the hen. "Please be good enough to leave **me** in peace, and **I** have no fear but **I** shall soon be well." Moral: Uninvited guests are often most welcome when **they** are gone ("The Cat and the Hen," Grosset & Dunlap, 1947, p. 133).

In passage 26, circle all of the *articles*:

26. Starting in **the** 1870s, another upheaval in **the** arts resulted from **the** development of **a** new approach to painting called Impressionism. Young artists rejected **the** long-accepted, conventional ways of presenting reality. They too were fascinated by recent discoveries in science and experimented with new techniques for capturing **the** effects of light. Often they used tiny dabs of complementary colors, relying on **the** viewer's eyes and mind to bring them together and form **the** desired effect. **The** Postimpressionist painters of **the** late nineteenth and early twentieth centuries worked out new ways of seeing that were highly personal. They scorned **the** old emphasis on reproducing reality as accurately as possible. Instead, they sought to express their own innermost visions and emotions (Harris, 1989, pp. 173–175).

In passages 27–28, circle all of the *conjunctions*:

27. A woman of many gifts, Margaret Fuller (1810–1850) is most aptly remembered **as** America's first true feminist. In her brief **yet** fruitful life, she was variously author, editor, literary **and** social critic, journalist, poet, **and** revolutionary. She was also one of the few female members of the prestigious Transcendentalist movement, whose ranks included Ralph Waldo Emerson, Henry David Thoreau, Elizabeth Palmer Peabody, Nathaniel Hawthorne, **and** many other prominent New England intellectuals of the day. **As** coeditor of the transcendentalist journal, *The Dial*, Fuller was able to give voice to her groundbreaking social critique on woman's place in society, the genesis of the book that was later to become *Woman in the Nineteenth Century* (Pine, 1999, p. 133).

28. **When** people started to analyze English grammar in the eighteenth century, it seemed logical to look at the language using the terms **and** distinctions which had proved so useful in studying Latin. English had no word-endings, it seemed. **Therefore**, it had no "grammar." **But** of course there is far more to grammar **than** word-endings. Some languages (such as Chinese) have none at all. English has less than a dozen types of regular endings (**and** a few irregular ones; Crystal, 2002, p. 22).

Exercise 10–2. Word Classes

For each word that is in bold, indicate its class—noun, pronoun, verb, adjective, adverb, conjunction, or preposition. Write the word next to the class on the lines following the passage:

Many trees **on** campus are not **native to** the **local** area. Eugene can **support** a greater **variety** of trees than many **places because its climate** is **moderate** enough to **easily** accommodate **trees** from colder **and** warmer **areas**. This **led** to the **campus** becoming an **arboretum**. However, planting nonnative trees **displaces** local trees. For **future** tree selections on campus, a **stronger emphasis** on native **species** would **eventually** turn the campus **into** a **richer learning environment**. One student commented **thoughtfully** that **her favorite** tree was the **Eastern black walnut**, near Gerlinger Hall.

Nouns (11):	variety, places, climate, trees, areas, campus, arboretum, emphasis, species, environment, walnut
Pronouns (2):	its, her
Verbs (3):	support, led, displaces
Adjectives (10):	native, local, moderate, future, stronger, richer, learning, favorite, Eastern, black
Adverbs (3):	easily, eventually, thoughtfully
Conjunctions (2):	because, and
Prepositions (3):	on, to, into

Exercise 10–3. Pronouns

1. Circle the *reflexive* pronouns: me   you   us   we   **ourselves**   him   her   **himself**

2. Circle the *demonstrative* pronouns: the   it   **that**   **those**   **these**   their   **this**

3. Circle the *interrogative* pronouns: he   on   under   **what**   her   **who**   **why**   must

4. Circle the *possessive* pronouns: **her**   that   **his**   **their**   any   only   ourselves

5. Circle the *relative* pronouns: **who**   his   **that**   their   **which**   them   they

Exercise 10–4. Particles Versus Prepositions

Circle the *particles*:

1. She threw **down** the pen.

2. He ran down the hill.

3. They sat on the bench.

4. He filled **up** his plate.

5. She ran to the door.

6. He took **off** the brace.

Circle the *prepositions*:

7. He gave away his books

8. She sat **by** the river.

9. They moved **to** Portland.

10. He ate **with** a fork.

11. She looked **at** the sea.

12. He ran **from** the dog.

Exercise 10–5. Adverbs

1. Circle the adverbs of *manner*: **quietly** **happily** somewhere forever dreamy

2. Circle the adverbs of *time*: **later** pleasantly lonely **now** everyone **always**

3. Circle the adverbs of *place*: **wherever** whenever forever **somewhere** **anywhere**

4. Circle the adverbs of *magnitude*: gleefully definitely **unusually** **slightly**

5. Circle the adverbs of *likelihood*: **possibly** joyously **probably** cleverly

Exercise 10–6. Conjunctions

1. Circle the *subordinate* conjunctions: forever   anyway   **unless**
   while   **before**

2. Circle the *coordinate* conjunctions: **and**   until   whenever   why
   to   **but**   off

3. Circle the *adverbial* conjuncts: **consequently**   because   while
   wherever   **thus**   **moreover**

Exercise 10–7. Review: Word Classes

Read the following fable. Then identify each type of word listed below by filling in the blanks. List each word only once.

The Lion and the Mouse

A lion was asleep in his den one day, when a mischievous mouse for no reason at all ran across the outstretched paw and up the royal nose of the king of beasts, awakening him from his nap. The mighty beast clapped his paw upon the now thoroughly frightened little creature and would have made an end of him.

"Please," squealed the mouse, "don't kill me. Forgive me this time, O King, and I shall never forget it. A day may come, who knows, when I may do you a good turn to repay your kindness." The lion, smiling at his little prisoner's fright and amused by the thought that so small a creature ever could be of assistance to the king of beasts, let him go.

Not long afterward the lion, while ranging the forest for his prey, was caught in the net which the hunters had set to catch him. He let out a roar that echoed through the forest. Even the mouse heard it, and recognizing the voice of his former preserver and friend, ran to the spot where he lay tangled in the net of ropes.

"Well, your majesty," said the mouse, "I know you did not believe me once when I said I would return a kindness, but here is my chance." And without further ado he set to work to nibble with his sharp little teeth at the ropes that bound the lion. Soon the lion was able to crawl out of the hunter's snare and be free.

Application: No act of kindness, no matter how small, is ever wasted.

Proverb: One good turn deserves another (Grosset & Dunlap, 1947, pp. 137–138).

List each type of word (list each word only once):

1. List the *nouns*: lion, den, day, mouse, reason, paw, nose, king, beasts, nap, creature, end, time, turn, kindness, fright, thought, assistance, forest, prey, net, hunters, roar, voice, preserver, friend, spot, ropes, majesty, chance, ado, teeth, snare, act, matter

2. List the *adjectives* (but not the participles): asleep, one, mischievous, royal, mighty, little, good, prisoner's, small, former, further, sharp, hunter's, free

3. List the *participles*: outstretched, awakening, frightened, smiling, amused, ranging, recognizing, tangled, wasted

4. List the *verbs*: was, ran, clapped, would have made, squealed, do kill, forgive, shall forget, may come, knows, may do, to repay, could be, let go, was caught, had set, to catch, let, echoed, heard, ran, lay, said, know, did believe, would return, is, set, to work, to nibble, bound, able to crawl, be, deserves

5. List the *adverbs*: now, thoroughly, never, so (small), ever, afterward, once, soon

Exercise 10–8 Phrases

In each sentence below, indicate the type of phrase that is bolded. Use the following codes:

NP = noun phrase

VP = verb phrase

PP = prepositional phrase

AJP = adjective phrase

AVP = adverb phrase

PP   1. The ball rolled **under the apple tree**.

AVP   2. The ranger told the ghost story **quite enthusiastically** to the teenagers.

VP   3. The hikers **had not yet arrived** back at camp by nightfall.

AVP   4. The two friends sat down together **very cheerfully** to enjoy their dinner.

NP   5. **The charming old village** overlooked the river.

AVP   6. Marty missed school **because of a stomach ache**.

VP   7. They **may have eaten** fish tonight for dinner.

PP   8. The resort specializes **in outdoor entertainment**.

VP   9. The lion **had been watching** the sparrows peck at the corn cobs.

NP   10. **The dry, old bread crumbs** had been left by a group of picnickers.

AVP   11. **Ever since Christmas**, Eva has been happy.

AJP   12. There are **several year-round, modernized, and attractive** inns in town.

NP   13. **Magnetic and electrical fields** may be present.

PP   14. The French have a holiday entitlement **of five weeks a year**.

AJP   15. There are **many long, steep, and winding** stretches of trail nearby.

NP   16. **The well-trained and persistent geologists** discovered large ice crystals.

AVP 17. The actor, tired and sick, struggled **rather mightily** to remember his lines.

AJP 18. The **densely wooded mountain** side was a familiar friend to all.

VP 19. Two crows **were fighting furiously** in the old corn field.

AJP 20. The poem was written in **flowery Victorian** language.

AVP 21. The children knocked on their new neighbor's door **somewhat shyly**.

VP 22. The athletes **were running** around the track to warm up before the meet.

AVP 23. **Before the race**, she double-knotted her track shoes.

AJP 24. Jimmy was thrilled with the **brand new, shiny, red** bicycle.

NP 25. **The rain-soaked graduation picnic** was a memorable event.

Exercise 10–9. Verb Tenses

For each of the sentences below, indicate the *verb tense* from the following choices:

A. Past perfect tense

B. Future progressive tense

C. Simple past tense

D. Present perfect tense

E. Simple future tense

F. Past progressive tense

G. Simple present tense

H. Present progressive tense

I. Future perfect tense

C 1. Yesterday, the Jones family arrived at Heathrow Airport around 2:00 p.m.

A 2. The direct flight from San Francisco had taken over 11 hours.

F 3. By 4:00 p.m., they were checking into their hotel in London.

F 4. Understandably, by early evening, all were feeling tired and hungry.

C 5. So they went out to a nearby pub for a delicious dinner of fish and chips.

A 6. By nine o'clock that evening, the family had settled into their room for the night.

G 7. It is now six o'clock in the morning, their first full day in the UK.

B 8. Today, the travelers will be taking the train from England to Wales.

I 9. They will have reached Llandudno, their final destination, by 11:30 a.m..

H 10. Now on the train, their son Liam is playing chess with his sister Jessie.

E 11. Jessie will eventually win the match, much to Liam's chagrin.

D 12. The children's mother, Martha, has just finished reading a short story.

H 13. And their father, Bruce, is ordering coffee from the trolley cart.

B 14. By two o'clock this afternoon, the Jones family will be enjoying the beach.

I 15. By that time, Liam will have forgotten about his loss to Jessie.

B 16. And Jessie will be searching for sea shells and colorful rocks.

D 17. Liam has just learned the Welsh name for Wales, "Cymu."

G 18. Suddenly, Jessie wants a red tee shirt with "Cymu" on the front.

E 19. Dad will buy it for her and one for Liam, too.

B 20. Soon the Jones family will be walking back to their B & B after a fun-filled day.

ANSWERS FOR CHAPTER 11: TYPES OF CLAUSES

Exercise 11–1

For the following sets of proverbs, fill in the clause type, using the following codes.

MC = main clause	INF = infinitive clause
REL = relative clause	PRT = participial clause
ADV = adverbial clause	GER = gerundive clause
NOM = nominal clause	

(Sources: *Category: Proverbs*, http://www.en.wikiquote.org/wiki/; *Creative proverbs from around the world*, http://www.creativeproverbs.com); Politis, Reich, & Sheldon, 1998; Scheffler, 1997; Stewart, 1997; Williams, 2000)

African Proverbs

1. A cutting word is **[MC]** worse than a bowstring. A cut may heal **[MC]**, but the cut of the tongue does **[MC]** not.

2. Ashes fly **[MC]** back into the face of him who throws **[REL]** them.

3. He who is being carried **[REL]** does not realize **[MC]** how far the town is **[NOM]**.

4. Quarrels end **[MC]** but words once spoken never die **[MC]**.

5. Send **[MC]** a boy where he wants **[ADV]** to go **[INF]** and you see **[MC]** his best pace.

6. Smooth seas do not make **[MC]** skillful sailors.

7. The lion does not turn **[MC]** around when a small dog barks **[ADV]**.

8. Two birds disputed **[MC]** about a kernel, when a third swooped **[ADV]** down and carried **[ADV]** it off.

9. When a needle falls **[ADV]** into a deep well, many people will look **[MC]** into the well, but few will be **[MC]** ready to go **[INF]** down after it.

10. He who learns **[REL]** teaches **[MC]**.

Chinese Proverbs

11. A bit of fragrance clings **[MC]** to the hand that gives **[REL]** flowers.

12. Even a hare will bite **[MC]** when it is **[ADV]** cornered.

13. A good fortune may forebode **[MC]** a bad luck, which may in turn disguise **[REL]** a good fortune.

14. If you are **[ADV]** patient in a moment of anger, you will escape **[MC]** a hundred days of sorrow.

15. If you do not study **[ADV]** hard when young, you'll end **[MC]** up bewailing **[PRT]** your failures as you grow up **[ADV]**.

16. Learning is **[MC]** a treasure that will follow **[REL]** its owner everywhere.

17. Listen **[MC]** to all, plucking **[PRT]** a feather from every passing goose, but follow **[MC]** no one absolutely.

18. Make **[MC]** happy those who are **[REL]** near, and those who are **[REL]** far will come **[MC]**.

19. Only when all contribute **[ADV]** their firewood can they build **[MC]** up a strong fire.

20. To attract **[INF]** good fortune, spend **[MC]** a new coin on an old friend, share **[MC]** an old pleasure with a new friend, and lift **[MC]** up the heart of a true friend by writing **[GER]** his name on the wings of a dragon.

Danish Proverbs

21. It is **[MC]** better to ask **[INF]** twice than to lose **[INF]** your way once.

22. He who builds **[REL]** according to every man's advice will have **[MC]** a crooked house.

23. Even a small star shines **[MC]** in the darkness.

24. A slip of the foot may soon be **[MC]** recovered, but that of the tongue perhaps never.

25. Kind words don't wear **[MC]** out the tongue.

26. Bad is **[MC]** never good until worse happens **[ADV]**.

27. Let **[MC]** deeds match **[INF]** words.

28. Speaking **[GER]** silence is **[MC]** better than senseless speech.

29. It is **[MC]** easy to sit **[INF]** at the helm in fine weather.

30. A good plan today is **[MC]** better than a perfect plan tomorrow.

German Proverbs

31. A good conscience is **[MC]** a soft pillow.

32. A single penny fairly got **[PRT]** is **[MC]** worth a thousand that are **[REL]** not.

33. All are **[MC]** not asleep who have **[REL]** their eyes shut.

34. Be **[MC]** silent, or say **[MC]** something better than silence.

35. Could everything be **[ADV]** done twice, everything would be **[MC]** done better.

36. If you would have **[ADV]** the lamp burn, you must pour **[MC]** oil into it.

37. Instead of complaining **[PRT]** that the rosebush is **[NOM]** full of thorns, be **[MC]** happy that the thorn bush has **[NOM]** roses.

38. It is **[MC]** better to turn **[INF]** back than go **[INF]** astray.

39. It is **[MC]** not till the cow has lost **[ADV]** her tail, that she discovers **[NOM]** its value.

40. Small undertakings give **[MC]** great comfort.

Hebrew Proverbs

41. Admission by the defendant is **[MC]** worth a hundred witnesses.

42. Do not confine **[MC]** your children to your own learning, for they were born **[ADV]** in another time.

43. Happy is **[MC]** the generation where the great listen **[NOM]** to the small, for it follows **[MC]** that in such a generation the small will listen **[NOM]** to the great.

44. Opinions founded **[PRT]** on prejudice are always sustained **[MC]** with the greatest violence.

45. Promise **[MC]** little and do **[MC]** much.

46. Rivalry of scholars advances **[MC]** wisdom.

47. The kind man feeds **[MC]** his cat before sitting **[GER]** down to dinner.

48. Whoever teaches **[NOM]** his son teaches **[MC]** not only his son but also his son's son, and so on to the end of generations.

49. Who seeks **[NOM]** more than he needs **[REL]** hinders **[MC]** himself from enjoying **[GER]** what he has **[NOM]**.

50. Slander slays **[MC]** three persons: the speaker, the spoken to, and the spoken of.

Irish Proverbs

51. Don't crow **[MC]** until you're **[ADV]** out of the woods.

52. Many an honest heart beats **[MC]** under a ragged coat.

53. The thing that is **[REL]** bought dear is often sold **[MC]** cheap.

54. Every dog is **[MC]** bold on its own doorstep.

55. Distant hills look **[MC]** green.

56. All happy endings are **[MC]** beginnings as well.

57. Praise **[MC]** the young and they will blossom **[MC]**.

58. A handful of skill is **[MC]** better than a bagful of gold.

59. Time is **[MC]** a great storyteller.

60. It takes **[MC]** time to build **[INF]** castles.

Japanese Proverbs

61. A single arrow is easily broken **[MC]**, but not ten in a bundle.

62. If you understand **[ADV]** everything, you must be **[MC]** misinformed.

63. Laughter cannot bring **[MC]** back what anger has driven **[NOM]** away.

64. One who smiles **[REL]** rather than rages **[REL]** is **[MC]** always the stronger.

65. We are **[MC]** no more than candles burning **[PRT]** in the wind.

66. When you're **[ADV]** thirsty, it's **[MC]** too late to think **[INF]** about digging **[GER]** a well.

67. The bamboo that bends **[REL]** is **[MC]** stronger than the oak that resists **[REL]**.

68. If money be **[ADV]** not thy servant, it will be **[MC]** thy master.

69. If you believe **[ADV]** everything you read **[REL]**, better not read **[MC]**.

70. If you want **[ADV]** a thing done well, do **[MC]** it yourself.

Mexican Proverbs

71. Conversation is **[MC]** food for the soul.

72. One must learn **[MC]** how to lose **[INF]** before learning **[GER]** how to play **[INF]**.

73. Tell **[MC]** me who your friends are **[NOM]** and I'll tell **[MC]** you who you are **[NOM]**.

74. It's **[MC]** not the fault of the mouse, but of the one who offers **[REL]** him the cheese.

75. In youth we learn **[MC]**, in old age we understand **[MC]**.

76. Money is **[MC]** a good servant, but an evil master.

77. Lions believe **[MC]** that everyone shares **[NOM]** their state of mind.

78. It is **[MC]** not enough to know **[INF]** how to ride **[INF]**; you must also know **[MC]** how to fall **[INF]**.

79. He who lives **[REL]** with hope dies **[MC]** happy.

80. When the river sounds **[ADV]**, it's **[MC]** because it carries **[ADV]** water.

Russian Proverbs

81. If you travel **[ADV]** more slowly, you will get **[MC]** farther.

82. A word is **[MC]** not a sparrow. If it flies **[ADV]** away, you won't catch **[MC]** it.

83. Not everything that glitters **[REL]** is **[MC]** gold.

84. Once you've committed **[ADV]** yourself to move **[INF]**, don't say **[MC]** you are **[NOM]** not up to it.

85. Any fish is **[MC]** good if it is **[ADV]** on the hook.

86. All's **[MC]** well that ends **[REL]** well.

87. One who sits **[REL]** between two chairs may easily fall **[MC]** down.

88. You will reap **[MC]** what you will sow **[NOM]**.

89. We do not care **[MC]** of what we have **[NOM]**, but we cry **[MC]** when it is **[ADV]** lost.

90. It is **[MC]** good to be **[INF]** visiting, but it is **[MC]** better at home.

Scottish Proverbs

91. A tale never loses **[MC]** in the telling.

92. Take care **[MC]** of your pennies and your dollars will take care **[MC]** of themselves.

93. They that dance **[REL]** must pay **[MC]** the fiddler.

94. They that will not be counseled **[REL]** cannot be helped **[MC]**.

95. What may be **[NOM]** done at any time will be **[MC]** done at no time.

96. Willful waste makes **[MC]** woeful want.

97. They that sow **[REL]** the wind shall reap **[MC]** the whirlwind.

98. When the cup is **[ADV]** full, carry **[MC]** it even.

99. Confession is **[MC]** good for the soul.

100. Get **[MC]** bait while the tide is **[ADV]** out.

Exercise 11–2

For the following quotations, fill in the clause type, using the following codes.

MC = main clause   INF = infinitive clause

REL = relative clause   PRT = participial clause

ADV = adverbial clause   GER = gerundive clause

NOM = nominal clause

(Sources: Bachelder, 1965; Benardete, 1961; Burke, 1996; Charlton, 1994; Great Quotations, 1990; McLellan, 1996; Quotable Shakespeare, n.d.; Searls, 2009; Thankful Kids, 2009; Who Said?, 2003).

Set A

1. I took **[MC]** a speed-reading course and read **[MC]** *War and Peace* in 20 minutes. It's **[MC]** about Russia. (Woody Allen)

2. I was **[MC]** seldom able to see **[INF]** an opportunity until it had ceased **[ADV]** to be **[INF]** one. (Mark Twain)

3. I must say **[MC]** I find **[NOM]** television very educational. The minute somebody turns **[REL]** it on, I go **[MC]** to the library and read **[MC]** a good book. (Groucho Marx)

4. Extemporaneous speaking should be practiced **[MC]** and cultivated **[MC]**. It is **[MC]** the lawyer's avenue to the public. (Abraham Lincoln)

5. Books were **[MC]** my pass to personal freedom. I learned **[MC]** to read **[INF]** at age three, and I soon discovered **[MC]** there was **[NOM]** a whole world to conquer **[INF]** that went **[REL]** beyond our farm in Mississippi. (Oprah Winfrey)

6. Modern cynics and skeptics see **[MC]** no harm in paying **[GER]** those to whom they entrust **[REL]** the minds of their children a smaller wage than is **[NOM]** paid to those to whom they entrust **[REL]** the care of their plumbing. (John F. Kennedy)

7. It has been said **[MC]** of the world's history hitherto that might makes **[NOM]** right. It is **[MC]** for us and for our time to reverse **[INF]** the maxim and to say **[INF]** that right makes **[NOM]** might. (Abraham Lincoln)

8. Most of the luxuries, and many of the so-called comforts of life, are **[MC]** not only not indispensable, but positive hindrances to the elevation of mankind. With respect to luxuries and comforts, the wisest have ever lived **[MC]** a more simple and meager life than the poor. The ancient philosophers, Chinese, Hindoo, Persian, and Greek, were **[MC]** a class than which none has been **[REL]** poorer in outward riches, none so rich in inward. (Henry David Thoreau)

9. Upon the subject of education, not presuming to dictate **[INF]** any plan or system respecting **[PRT]** it, I can only say **[MC]** that I view **[NOM]** it as the most important subject which we as a people can be engaged **[REL]** in. That every man may receive **[NOM]** at least a moderate education, and thereby be **[INF]** enabled to read **[INF]** the histories of his own and other countries, by which he may duly appreciate **[ADV]** the value of our free institutions, appears **[MC]** to be **[INF]** an object of vital importance. (Abraham Lincoln)

10. I always wanted **[MC]** to be **[INF]** somebody, but I should have been **[MC]** more specific. (Lily Tomlin)

Set B

11. Once they notice **[ADV]** you, they never completely close **[MC]** the file. (Philip K. Dick).

12. I am **[NOM]** invisible, understand **[MC]**, simply because people refuse **[ADV]** to see **[INF]** me. (Ralph Ellison)

13. Freedom is **[MC]** indivisible. (Nelson Mandela)

14. But to live **[INF]** outside the law, you must be **[MC]** honest. (Bob Dylan)

15. It ain't **[MC]** over 'til it's **[ADV]** over. (Yogi Berra)

16. For the spectator even more than for the artist, art is **[MC]** a habit-forming drug. (Marcel Duchamp)

17. Though I am **[ADV]** in the depths of misery, there is **[MC]** still calmness, pure harmony, and music inside me. (Vincent van Gogh)

18. Never in the field of human conflict was **[MC]** so much owed **[PRT]** by so many to so few. (Winston Churchill)

19. Time spent **[PRT]** with a cat is **[MC]** never wasted. (Sydney Hauser)

20. Everybody talks **[MC]** about people, but nobody ever does **[MC]** anything about them. (Fran Lebowitz)

Set C

21. I want **[MC]** to bend **[INF]** this note, bend **[INF]** that note, sing **[INF]** this way, sing **[INF]** that way, and get **[INF]** all the feeling, eat **[INF]** all the good foods, and travel **[INF]** all over in one day, and you can't do **[MC]** it. (Billie Holiday)

22. Happy is **[MC]** the house that shelters **[REL]** a cat. (Sydney Hauser)

23. If I had **[ADV]** to sum **[INF]** up the totality of the Woodstock experience, I would say **[MC]** it was **[NOM]** the first attempt to land **[INF]** a man on the Earth. (Abbie Hoffman)

24. Never doubt **[MC]** that a small group of thoughtful, committed people can change **[NOM]** the world. (Margaret Mead)

25. Let **[MC]** them eat **[INF]** cake. (Marie-Antoinette)

26. To thine own self be **[MC]** true, and it must follow **[MC]**, as the night the day, thou canst not then be **[NOM]** false to any man. (William Shakespeare)

27. The future always looks **[MC]** good in the golden land, because no one remembers **[ADV]** the past. (Joan Didion)

28. In the attitude of silence, the soul finds **[MC]** the path in a clearer light, and what is **[NOM]** elusive and deceptive resolves **[MC]** itself into crystal clearness. (Mahatma Gandhi)

29. Half finished work generally proves **[MC]** to be **[INF]** labor lost. (Abraham Lincoln)

30. We have lived **[MC]** not in proportion to the number of years that we have spent **[REL]** on the earth, but in proportion as we have enjoyed **[ADV]**. (Henry David Thoreau)

Set D

31. Nothing so needs **[MC]** reforming as other people's habits. (Mark Twain)

32. Happiness lies **[MC]** in the joy of achievement and the thrill of creative effort. (Franklin D. Roosevelt)

33. Brevity is **[MC]** the soul of wit. (William Shakespeare)

34. Keep **[MC]** your face to the sunshine and you cannot see **[MC]** the shadow. (Helen Keller)

35. The time to repair **[INF]** the roof is **[MC]** when the sun is shining **[ADV]**. (John F. Kennedy)

36. The only way to get **[INF]** the best of an argument is **[MC]** to avoid **[INF]** it. (Dale Carnegie)

37. California is **[MC]** a Garden of Eden, a paradise to live **[INF]** in or see **[INF]**. (Woody Guthrie)

38. Fair is **[MC]** foul, and foul is **[MC]** fair. (William Shakespeare)

39. Be **[MC]** who you are **[NOM]** and say **[MC]** what you feel **[NOM]**. (Dr. Seuss)

40. All philosophers must soar **[MC]** with unwearied passion until they grasp **[ADV]** the true nature of things as they really are **[ADV]**. (Plato)

Set E

41. The young boy asked **[MC]**, "Why should I become **[NOM]** a scholar when I can make **[ADV]** more money in the market place?" Plato replied **[MC]** that, "the pursuit of wisdom and truth is **[NOM]** essential to our integrity as human beings."

42. Moving **[GER]** the ship of state is **[MC]** a slow process. States are **[MC]** like big tankers. They're **[MC]** not like speedboats. (Barack Obama)

43. Good leadership requires **[MC]** you to surround **[INF]** yourself with people of diverse perspectives who can disagree **[REL]** with you without fear of retaliation. (Doris Kearns Goodwin)

44. Sometimes leadership is **[MC]** planting **[GER]** trees under whose shade you'll never sit **[REL]**. (Jennifer M. Granholm)

45. It takes **[MC]** 20 years to build **[INF]** a reputation and five minutes to ruin **[INF]** it. If you think **[ADV]** about that, you'll do **[MC]** things differently. (Warren Buffett)

46. How wonderful it is **[MC]** that nobody need **[NOM]** wait **[INF]** a single moment before starting **[GER]** to improve **[INF]** the world. (Anne Frank)

47. Unless someone like you cares **[ADV]** a whole lot, nothing is going **[MC]** to get **[INF]** better. It's **[MC]** not. (Dr. Seuss)

48. With every good deed, you are sowing **[MC]** a seed, though the harvest you may not see **[ADV]**. (Anonymous)

49. The more we study **[REL]** the more we discover **[MC]** our ignorance. (Percy Bysshe Shelley)

50. My teacher helps **[MC]** me out a lot and she is **[MC]** nice to me and she teaches **[MC]** me about stuff and when I first came **[ADV]** to her classroom, I was **[MC]** afraid of bugs but now I'm **[MC]** not. (Krysten, age 8)

Set F

51. Education is **[MC]** what survives **[REL]** when what has been learned **[REL]** has been forgotten **[ADV]**. (B. F. Skinner)

52. My karate teacher can break **[MC]** 12 bats over his head and 10 bricks with his bare hands. (Billy, age 7)

53. My teacher is **[MC]** fun and hard-working and never forgets **[MC]** to take **[INF]** time to talk **[INF]** to her students, unlike some teachers who only teach **[REL]** and never talk **[REL]**. (Sarah, age 11)

54. The mystic chords of memory, stretching **[PRT]** from every battlefield, and patriot grave, to every living heart and hearthstone, all over this broad land, will yet swell **[MC]** the chorus of the Union, when again touched **[PRT]**, as surely they will be **[ADV]**, by the better angels of our nature. (Abraham Lincoln; Wilson, 2006, p. 67)

55. I remember **[MC]** when my second-grade teacher pushed **[NOM]** me and pushed me **[NOM]** to read **[INF]** and when I finally started **[ADV]** to read **[INF]**, I liked **[MC]** it so much I couldn't stop **[NOM]**! (Chris, age 8)

56. The art of teaching **[GER]** is **[MC]** the art of assisting **[GER]** discovery. (Mark Van Doren)

57. Human history becomes **[MC]** more and more a race between education and catastrophe. (H. G. Wells)

58. Leave **[MC]** it longer on top, so I can have **[ADV]** spikes. My mom wrote **[MC]** on the form, "no Mohawk," so I can't have **[MC]** that. (David, age 13)

59. I am **[MC]** thankful for my dad because he never yells **[ADV]** at me. (Victor, 2nd grade).

60. I'm **[MC]** thankful that the Ducks are going **[NOM]** to beat **[INF]** the Beavers. I'm **[MC]** thankful that I have **[NOM]** clothes to wear **[INF]** and parents who care **[REL]** about me. (Frankie, 7th grade)

Exercise 11–3

For the following fable, fill in the clause type, using the codes below.

MC = main clause   INF = infinitive clause

REL = relative clause   PRT = participial clause

ADV = adverbial clause   GER = gerundive clause

NOM = nominal clause

The Lion and the Mouse

A lion was **[MC]** asleep in his den one day, when a mischievous mouse for no reason at all ran **[ADV]** across the outstretched paw and up the royal nose of the king of beasts, awakening **[PRT]** him from his nap. The mighty beast clapped **[MC]** his paw upon the now thoroughly frightened little creature and would have made **[MC]** an end of him.

"Please," squealed **[MC]** the mouse, "don't kill **[NOM]** me. Forgive **[MC]** me this time, O King, and I shall never forget **[MC]** it. A day may come **[MC]**, who knows, when I may do **[NOM]** you a good turn to repay **[INF]** your kindness." The lion, smiling **[PRT]** at his little prisoner's fright and amused **[PRT]** by the thought that so small a creature ever could be **[REL]** of assistance to the king of beasts, let **[MC]** him go **[INF]**.

Not long afterward the lion, while ranging **[PRT]** the forest for his prey, was caught **[MC]** in the net which the hunters had set **[REL]** to catch **[INF]** him. He let **[MC]** out a roar that echoed **[REL]** through the forest. Even the mouse heard **[MC]** it, and recognizing **[PRT]** the voice of his former preserver and friend, ran **[MC]** to the spot where he lay **[REL]** tangled in the net of ropes.

"Well, your majesty," said **[MC]** the mouse, "I know **[NOM]** you did not believe **[NOM]** me once when I said **[ADV]** I would return **[NOM]** a kindness, but here is **[NOM]** my chance." And without further ado he set **[MC]** to work **[INF]** to nibble **[INF]** with his sharp little teeth at the ropes that bound **[REL]** the lion. Soon the lion was able **[MC]** to crawl **[INF]** out of the hunter's snare and be **[INF]** free.

Application: No act of kindness, no matter how small, is **[MC]** ever wasted.

Proverb: One good turn deserves **[MC]** another (Grosset & Dunlap, 1947, pp. 137–138).

Exercise 11–4. Coding Child and Adolescent Language Samples

The following exercises provide additional practice coding clauses in spoken or written language samples (or excerpts of samples) that were produced by children and adolescents. For each exercise, fill in the blanks using the following codes:

MC = main clause   INF = infinitive clause

REL = relative clause   PRT = participial clause

ADV = adverbial clause   GER = gerundive clause

NOM = nominal clause

#1: Judy, 11th grade (TLD) (from the author's files)

General Conversation Task:

1. I'm **[MC]** a junior.

2. I think **[MC]** I want **[NOM]** to go **[INF]** into the elementary educational field.

3. I like **[MC]** little kids.

4. I'm taking **[MC]** keyboarding, ITT which is **[REL]** international trade and tourism, and a cooking class called **[PRT]** world cooking.

5. And then I'm taking **[MC]** English.

6. And I have **[MC]** a worker's experience period where I go **[REL]** and work **[REL]** at my job (so).

7. I work **[MC]** for an insurance company right now.

8. So I work **[MC]** there doing **[PRT]** the filing.

9. It makes **[MC]** the car payment.

10. (So we get) So we already have **[MC]** college credit.

Favorite Game or Sport Task:

1. And there's **[MC]** foul balls, which means **[REL]** there's **[NOM]** lines drawn **[PRT]** from the home plate through the first base out to the field like to the fence like 180 feet.

2. And then there's **[MC]** a line drawn **[PRT]** from the third base line that goes **[REL]** out.

3. And if the ball goes **[ADV]** past the line to the left in the line not in the playing field, it's **[MC]** a foul ball.

4. And that's **[MC]** just a ball.

5. So (it) your count is **[MC]** still there.

6. And you have **[MC]** a count when you're **[ADV]** at bat.

7. And then (four balls or yeah) four balls means **[MC]** you walk **[NOM]**.

8. And so when you get **[ADV]** the base automatically, you can't make **[MC]** an out with that.

9. And then (the base runners) like if you're **[ADV]** on base, you can advance **[MC]** as soon as the ball leaves **[ADV]** the pitcher's hand.

10. And you can run **[MC]** the bases until you get **[ADV]** out or until your coach tells **[ADV]** you to stop **[INF]**.

Peer Conflict Resolution Task:

Examiner: What is a good way for Debbie to deal with Melanie?

1. Maybe if there's **[ADV]** a writing part, she can do **[MC]** the writing part and at least be **[MC]** there and help **[MC]** them and try **[MC]** to say **[INF]** what she feels **[NOM]** about the whole thing and see **[MC]** if she has **[NOM]** any advice of what they should do **[NOM]** better.

2. Or (like if just) basically have **[MC]** a session where they can just talk **[REL]** and (see what) split **[REL]** it up into teamwork, working wise.

Examiner: Why is that a good way for Debbie to deal with Melanie?

3. So she doesn't judge **[MC]** her.

4. Say **[MC]** she doesn't do **[NOM]** what she's supposed **[NOM]** to do **[INF]**.

5. But if she talks **[ADV]** to her and sees **[ADV]**, then maybe they can change **[MC]** some things.

6. So that will help **[MC]**.

Examiner: What do you think will happen if Debbie does that?

7. Well, she could either say **[MC]** "no" and ignore **[MC]** her.

8. Or she could say **[MC]** "yes."

9. And they could work **[MC]** the problem out.

10. But if she says **[ADV]** "no," then I guess **[MC]** she could go **[NOM]** to the teacher and see **[NOM]** what they could do **[NOM]** about it, see **[NOM]** if maybe she could get **[NOM]** another student to help **[INF]** them or have **[NOM]** more time so the two can just work **[ADV]** on it, Debbie and the other girl.

#2: *Saeda, 2nd grade* (Thankful Kids, 2009)

Expository Essay

I am **[MC]** thankful for trees because they make **[ADV]** oxygen for me, water because it will make **[ADV]** me not dehydrated, and books because when I read **[ADV]**, I can learn **[ADV]** and I love **[ADV]** to read.

#3: *Alex, 3rd grade* (Thankful Kids, 2009)

Expository Essay

These are **[MC]** some things I am **[REL]** thankful for. I'm **[MC]** thankful for my food, my lunch, and everything that is **[REL]** in it. I'm **[MC]** glad that it is **[NOM]** a good fruit. I'm **[MC]** thankful for all the water and milk that we have **[REL]**. I'm **[MC]** thankful for my house. My house is **[MC]** warm and cozy. I love **[MC]** my house so much. My house is **[MC]** special. I am **[MC]** thankful for my school. I'm **[MC]** so thankful for my teacher. I'm **[MC]** thankful for all the recess we get **[REL]**. I'm **[MC]** thankful for my special book. I'm **[MC]** so lucky for all these things.

#4: *Kyra, 5th grade* (Thankful Kids, 2009)

Expository Essay

I'm **[MC]** so thankful for my pets to be **[INF]** a part of my family. Every single day, I wake up **[MC]** with warmth on my legs from my dog Toby sleeping **[PRT]** on my legs. When Toby hears **[ADV]** my bus, he will wait **[MC]** at the door until I come **[ADV]** home. Right when Toby sees **[ADV]** me, he will lick **[MC]** me until I can't feel **[ADV]** my face and all I can taste **[REL]** is **[ADV]** slobber. I am **[MC]** so happy and thankful to have **[INF]** a dog like Toby.

#5: *Paris, 7th grade* (Thankful Kids, 2009)

Expository Essay

I am **[MC]** very thankful to have **[INF]** a mom that can be **[REL]** around me, even if I don't always want **[ADV]** her around. She comforts

[MC] me when I'm [ADV] sad or sick. She helps [MC] me through the bad times. She cooks [MC] and provides [MC] for me even if there's [ADV] barely anything in the bank. She is [MC] my mother. And her name is [MC] Pam. But don't you wear [MC] it out. That's [MC] my job. I'm [MC] very thankful for a mother that cares [REL].

#6: Roberto, 8th grade (Thankful Kids, 2009)

Letter to a Former Teacher

There are [MC] many people in my life for whom I'm [REL] thankful for. But you are [MC] the only person that comes [REL] to mind when I think [ADV] of it. Through help and guidance, you are [MC] the one who helped [REL] me through sixth grade. I remember [MC] when you gave [NOM] me the Honor Society application sheet. You told [MC] me to get [INF] every teacher to sign [INF] my recommendation sheets and to write [INF] the essay to tell [INF] why I should be [NOM] in the Honor Society. You made [MC] sure that I got [NOM] my essay done and my recommendation sheets in. You made [MC] sure I was doing [NOM] it because you knew [ADV] that I would have [NOM] a chance to be [INF] in the Honor Society. I truly believe [MC] that without you, I would have never gotten [NOM] to where I am [ADV] today. I will never forget [MC] the things you did [REL] for me. And that's [MC] why I wanted [NOM] to say [INF], "Thank you."

#7: Emily, 3rd grade (TLD) (from the author's files)

Narrative Essay: "The Swan"

Once upon a time, there was [MC] a swan. She was going [MC] to have [INF] some babies. But she had never had [MC] babies before. She was [MC] nervous! So she asked [MC] the falcon for some advice. But *she* [the falcon] was asking [MC] that same question. So they went [MC] to look [INF] for someone to help [INF] them. So they asked [MC] the raven for her advice. She said [MC], "Ask [NOM] the ostrich. She knows [NOM]." They went [MC] to the ostrich. She said [MC] she thought [NOM] and thought **[NOM]**. At last, she said **[MC]**, "Why don't you try **[NOM]** laying **[GER]** on the nest and wait **[NOM]** a while. And they will hatch **[MC]**. That's **[MC]** what I would do **[NOM]**." So they went **[MC]** to their nests and sat **[MC]** and sat **[MC]**. And then they said **[MC]**, "I feel **[NOM]** something wiggling." "It must be **[NOM]** the babies," said **[MC]** the swan and raven. And that was **[MC]** it. And of course they were **[MC]** very excited. The end.

#8: *Ryan, 5th grade (TLD)* (from the author's files)

Expository Essay: The Nature of Friendship

Do you have **[MC]** a friend? I do **[MC]**. What do you think **[MC]** friendship means **[NOM]**? I think **[MC]** it means **[NOM]** someone you can trust **[REL]**, someone you can depend **[REL]** on, someone you have **[REL]** a lot in common with, and somebody who keeps **[REL]** secrets. Sometimes people feel **[MC]** lonely and have **[MC]** no one to talk **[INF]** to. That can lead **[MC]** to sadness. That is **[MC]** some reasons why friendship is **[NOM]** important. Sometimes friendship comforts **[MC]** you and makes **[MC]** you feel **[INF]** less alone. Me and my friends like **[MC]** to play **[INF]** lots and lots of video games together. Some advice for good friendship is **[MC]** to not annoy **[INF]** the person, be **[INF]** nice to the person. Do not tell **[MC]** secrets that they have told **[REL]** you.

#9: *Mark, 8th grade (TLD)* (from the author's files)

Expository Essay: The Nature of Friendship

Friendship is **[MC]** basically an understanding between two people who share **[REL]** common interests or beliefs. Friendship is **[MC]** about being **[GER]** able to trust **[INF]** that person and being **[GER]** able to spend **[INF]** time with them. Friendship is **[MC]** important to people because it gives **[ADV]** them a chance to do **[INF]** things that they like **[REL]** with someone they enjoy **[REL]** spending **[GER]** time with. Having **[GER]** friends makes **[MC]** life more enjoyable because you have **[ADV]** someone you can talk **[REL]** to and that you like **[REL]** to do **[INF]** things with. Friends do **[MC]** all kinds of things together from going **[GER]** on hikes to going **[GER]** to the movies. Friends can talk **[MC]** to each other and go **[MC]** places together. People who generally become **[REL]** friends are **[MC]** those who have **[REL]** common interests. If someone had **[ADV]** completely different opinions about what is **[NOM]** fun to do **[INF]** than someone else, then they probably won't become **[MC]** very good friends. The kinds of things that can harm **[REL]** a friendship are **[MC]** things like arguing **[GER]** and fighting **[GER]**. If you intentionally do **[ADV]** something that you know **[REL]** they won't like **[REL]**, it will damage **[MC]** a friendship. A way to maintain **[INF]** a friendship is **[MC]** to continually spend **[INF]** time with them. That way you can still talk **[MC]** to each other even if they live **[ADV]** a long ways away. That can help **[MC]** people remain **[INF]** friends. There are **[MC]** always ways to maintain **[INF]** friendships. Sometimes it is **[MC]** just hard to figure **[INF]** out how.

#10: Willow, 8th grade (Teachers Need to Be Healthy, 2009)

Letter to the Editor (Persuasive Essay)

We think **[MC]** that the ban of junk foods in schools should include **[NOM]** teachers. Sodas and other junk foods are **[MC]** just as unhealthy for teachers as they are **[ADV]** for students. The teachers need **[MC]** to set **[INF]** a good example for the students. If students see **[ADV]** that the ban on junk food includes **[NOM]** teachers as well as themselves, they might be **[MC]** more willing to go **[INF]** along with the ban. To have **[INF]** a mind and body that functions **[REL]** the best they can **[REL]**, you need **[MC]** to eat **[INF]** the proper amount of nutrients. You do not get **[MC]** these nutrients from junk foods and soda. Because of this, you do not function **[MC]** as well as you could **[ADV]**. We think **[MC]** it is **[NOM]** important for teachers to have **[INF]** healthy bodies and minds, so that they will teach **[ADV]** the students better than otherwise. If teachers eat or drink **[ADV]** junk food or soda, they will not teach **[MC]** as well. If the teachers really cannot live **[ADV]** without the junk food, they can very easily just eat **[MC]** it at their homes. It should not be **[MC]** that hard for them to wait **[INF]** the seven or eight hours that their jobs take **[REL]** up to eat **[INF]** junk food if they need **[ADV]** it that badly. After all, students can **[MC]**.

#11: *Trevor, 5th grade (TLD)* (from the author's files)

Persuasive Essay: The Circus Controversy

I think **[MC]** it is **[NOM]** a bad idea to have **[INF]** animals in the circus because animals should be **[ADV]** free to do **[INF]** what they want **[NOM]**. They're **[MC]** stuck in small cages. So there is **[MC]** barely enough room to get **[INF]** their adequate exercise. People don't like **[MC]** to be **[INF]** imprisoned. So we should let **[MC]** them go **[INF]**. Then they won't be **[MC]** forced to do **[INF]** tricks. I think **[MC]** it is **[NOM]** cruel to train **[INF]** animals to do **[INF]** a trick because if they don't do **[ADV]** it right, the trainers will hit **[ADV]** them. These are **[MC]** the reasons why I think **[NOM]** circuses should not be **[NOM]** allowed. For the animals' sake.

#12: *Carl, 11th grade (TLD)* (from the author's files)

Persuasive Essay: The Circus Controversy

A common controversy is **[MC]** often whether or not circuses are **[NOM]** good or bad for the community. I like **[MC]** the clowns because often times they are **[ADV]** also animal trainers. However, there is **[MC]** a downside to all these beneficial factors. Frequently, the animals are **[MC]** underfed and are kept **[MC]** in small cages. This alone infuriates **[MC]** animal enthusiasts everywhere. Circuses can be **[MC]** cruel to animals. Therefore, they should be closed **[MC]** down. If animals feel **[ADV]** threatened, they could be **[MC]** dangerous when they fight **[ADV]** back. What I believe **[NOM]** is **[MC]** that a circus could hire **[NOM]** more people and have them go **[INF]** to clown school. Everybody likes **[MC]** clowns, right? The hardest part of this would be **[MC]** training **[GER]** all those clowns. Still, with a little creativity and some ingenuity, I think **[MC]** a clown school could be **[NOM]** possible. Overall, I think **[MC]** animals should not be **[NOM]** in circuses.

ANSWERS FOR CHAPTER 12: TYPES OF SENTENCES

Exercise 12–1

For each quotation, indicate whether the sentence is:

A. Simple   C. Compound
B. Complex   D. Compound-complex

1. __B__ All philosophers must soar with unwearied passion until they grasp the true nature of things as they really are. (Plato)

2. __B__ Education is not filling a pail but the lighting of a fire. (William Butler Yeats)

3. __B__ If you bungle raising your children, I don't think whatever else you do well matters very much. (Jacqueline Kennedy Onassis)

4. __A__ A little learning is a dangerous thing. (Alexander Pope)

5. __C__ Never give up and never give in. (Hubert H. Humphrey)

6. __A__ Life is a festival only to the wise. (Ralph Waldo Emerson)

7. __B__ No one can make you feel inferior without your consent. (Eleanor Roosevelt)

8. __B__ To talk in public, to think in solitude, to read and to hear, to inquire and answer inquiries, is the business of the scholar. (Samuel Johnson)

9. __B__ My teacher is special because she never yells at me. (Rebecca, age 8)

10. __B__ There's something about taking a plow and breaking new ground. (Ken Kesey)

11. __B__ The more we study, the more we discover our ignorance. (Percy Bysshe Shelley)

12. __D__ My teacher helps me out a lot and she is nice to me and she teaches me about stuff and when I first came to her classroom, I was afraid of bugs but now I'm not. (Krysten, age 8)

13. __B__ Education is what survives when what has been learned has been forgotten. (B. F. Skinner)

14. __A__ My karate teacher can break 12 bats over his head and 10 bricks with his bare hands. (Billy, age 7)

15. __D__ My teacher is fun and hard-working and never forgets to take time to talk to her students, unlike some teachers who only teach and never talk. (Sarah, age 11)

16. __A__ Mix with your sage counsels some brief folly. (Cicero)

17. __D__ I remember when my second-grade teacher pushed me and pushed me to read and when I finally started to read, I liked it so much I couldn't stop! (Chris, age 8)

18. __B__ The art of teaching is the art of assisting discovery. (Mark Van Doren)

19. __B__ Leave it longer on top, so I can have spikes. (David, age 13)

20. __C__ My mom wrote on the form, "no Mohawk," so I can't get that. (David, age 13)

Exercise 12–2. Hierarchical Complexity

For each of the following sentences, indicate the number of levels of embedding it contains. Begin by coding each sentence for each type of clause it contains:

MC = main clause   INF = infinitive clause

ADV = adverbial clause   PRT = participial clause

NOM = nominal clause   GER = gerundive clause

REL = relative clause

1. Even if you're **[ADV]** on the right track, you'll get run **[MC]** over if you just sit **[ADV]** there.   Levels: 1

2. With every good deed, you are sowing **[MC]** a seed, though the harvest you may not see **[ADV]**.   Levels: 1

3. Use **[MC]** a small paintbrush and a paper cup with the smaller beetles because you can damage **[ADV]** them if you pick **[ADV]** them up in your hand.   Levels: 2

4. Jason's little sister Amanda has **[MC]** an ear infection for which her pediatrician prescribed **[REL]** a liquid antibiotic that must be kept **[REL]** refrigerated.   Levels: 2

5. Every miler knows **[MC]**, in the way a sailor knows **[REL]** the middle of the ocean, that it is **[NOM]** not the first lap but the third that is **[REL]** farthest from the finish line. (Parker, 2009, p. 246)   Levels: 2

6. As Jim and I went **[ADV]** over to see **[INF]** what was going **[NOM]** on, someone crawled **[MC]** out of the closet. (Boy, age 13)   Levels: 3

7. Before you take **[ADV]** a piece, like if there was **[ADV]** a rook right here, you kind of make **[MC]** sure because there is **[ADV]** a strategy that you can do **[REL]** to try **[INF]** to get **[INF]** a king in checkmate with two rooks. (Boy, age 11)   Levels: 4

8. I hated **[MC]** him on sight and sound and would be **[MC]** about to put **[INF]** my dog whistle to my lips and blow **[INF]** him off the face of Christmas when suddenly he, with a violet wink, put **[ADV]** *his* whistle to *his* lips and blew **[ADV]** so stridently, so high, so exquisitely loud, that gobbling faces, their cheeks bulged **[PRT]** with goose, would press **[NOM]** against their tinseled windows, the whole length of the white echoing street. (Thomas, 1954, p. 22)   Levels: 3

Exercise 12–3

Code the following sentences. Then rewrite each sentence in the active voice and code it again.

1. It was promised **[MC]** by Mozart that the duets would be completed **[NOM]** soon.

   Active: Mozart promised **[MC]** that he would complete **[NOM]** the duets soon.

2. The missing duets, which had been misplaced **[REL]** by Frederick, were presented **[MC]** by Mozart to his friend Joseph Haydn.

   Active: Mozart presented **[MC]** the missing duets, which Frederick had misplaced **[REL]**, to his friend Joseph Haydn.

3. It was known **[MC]** by all patrons that a symphony could be written **[NOM]** by Mozart in minutes.

    Active: All patrons knew **[MC]** that Mozart could write **[NOM]** a symphony in minutes.

4. An amazing tonal richness was achieved **[MC]** by the string quartet, which was led **[REL]** by a new cellist from Philadelphia.

    Active: The string quartet achieved **[MC]** an amazing tonal richness under the leadership of a new cellist from Philadelphia.

    OR: The new cellist from Philadelphia led **[MC]** the string quartet as it achieved **[ADV]** an amazing tonal richness.

5. The miniature trio for three strings was created **[MC]** by the new composer who was paid **[REL]** handsomely by the king's court.

    Active: The new composer created **[MC]** the miniature trio for three strings, and the king's court paid **[MC]** him/her handsomely.

    OR: The new composer, whom the king's court paid **[REL]** handsomely, created **[MC]** the miniature trio for three strings.

6. The young musician was supported **[MC]** by a generous scholarship funded **[PRT]** by a wealthy elderly patron, to attend **[INF]** the Juilliard School of Music.

    Active: A wealthy elderly patron funded **[MC]** a generous scholarship to support **[INF]** the young musician so that he/she could attend **[ADV]** the Juilliard School of Music.

7. The composer's status of nobility was implied **[MC]** by the "von" inserted **[PRT]** before his last name, which was preferred **[REL]** by some over the plainer "Ernst Dohnanyi."

    Active: The "von" that was inserted **[REL]** before his last name implied **[MC]** the composer's status of nobility, which some people preferred **[REL]** over the plainer "Ernst Dohnanyi."

8. The flute quartet was performed **[MC]** by four young musicians who had been hired **[REL]** by a royal family to educate **[INF]** its children in the finer things in life.

   Active: To educate **[INF]** its children in the finer things of life, the royal family hired **[MC]** four young musicians who played **[REL]** the flute quartet.

9. A dramatic conclusion to the Christmas play was anticipated **[MC]** by members of the audience, many of whom had been coerced **[REL]** into attending **[GER]** the performance.

   Active: Members of the audience anticipated **[MC]** a dramatic conclusion to the Christmas play because someone had coerced **[ADV]** many of them into attending **[GER]** the performance.

10. The rock concert, sold out **[PRT]** for months, had to be cancelled **[MC]** by the vendor because the band's lead singer had been delayed **[ADV]** by inclement weather in Chicago.

    Active: The vendor had to cancel **[MC]** the rock concert, which had been sold out **[REL]** for months, because inclement weather in Chicago delayed **[ADV]** the band's lead singer.

ANSWERS FOR CHAPTER 13: UNITS OF MEASUREMENT

Exercise 13–1. Identifying T-units

For each of the following paragraphs, indicate with a slash (/) the end of each T-unit:

1. Once Oregon was thought to be immune to earthquakes / today we know that we have them in three different flavors—devastating subduction earthquakes like the 1700 catastrophe, deep intraplate earthquakes like the Puget_Sound temblors of 1949 and 2001, and sharp local jolts like the Spring_Break_Quake of 1993 / (Sullivan, 2008, p. 67)

   > How many T-units are contained in this paragraph?   2
   >
   > How many words did Sullivan use?   47
   >
   > What is Sullivan's MLTU?   23.50
   >
   > How many of Sullivan's T-units are complex sentences?   2

2. Beatrix_Potter was a Londoner, born there in 1866 / but her family had connections with Lancashire cotton / and she spent her holidays from the age of 16 in the Lake_District, in rented, but rather grand houses, round Windermere and Derwentwater / her parents were genteel, upper middle class Edwardians / and she was educated at home and expected to devote her life to her parents or get married / she found an outlet for artistic talents in drawing and painting "little books for children" / and encouraged by the family's Lakeland friend, Canon_Rawnsley, her first book, *Peter_Rabbit*, was published in 1901 / (Davies, 1989, p. 179)

   > How many T-units are contained in this paragraph?   7
   >
   > How many words did Davies use?   96
   >
   > What is Davies' MLTU?   13.71
   >
   > How many T-units are complex sentences?   4

3. I have become a little more skillful in guessing right explanations and in devising experimental tests / but this may probably be the result of mere practice, and of a larger store of knowledge / I have as much difficulty as ever in expressing myself clearly and concisely / and this difficulty has caused me a very great loss of time / but it has had the compensating advantage of forcing me to think long and intently about every sentence / and thus I have been often led to see errors in reasoning and in my own observations or those of others / (Charles Darwin, 1958, pp. 136–137)

How many T-units are contained in this paragraph?   6

How many words did Darwin use?   97

What is Darwin's MLTU?   16.17

How many of Darwin's T-units are complex sentences?   4

4. Some birds, such as most eagles, hawks, ospreys, falcons, and vultures, migrate during the day / larger birds can hold more body fat, go longer without eating, and take longer to migrate / these birds glide along on rising columns of warm air, called thermals, which hold them aloft while they slowly make their way north or south / they generally rest at night and hunt early in the morning before the sun has a chance to warm up the land and create good soaring conditions / birds migrating during the day use a combination of landforms, rivers, and the rising and setting sun to guide them in the right direction / (Tekiela, 2001, p. xv)

How many T-units are contained in this paragraph?   5

How many words did Tekiela use?   107

What is Tekiela's MLTU?   21.40

How many of Tekiela's T-units are complex sentences?   4

5. In the morning I watched the geese from the door through the mist, sailing in the middle of the pond, fifty rods off, so large and tumultuous that Walden appeared like an artificial pond for their

amusement / but when I stood on the shore they at once rose up with a great flapping of wings at the signal of their commander, and when they had got into rank circled about over my head, twenty_nine of them, and then steered straight to Canada, with a regular *honk* from the leader at intervals, trusting to break their fast in muddier pools / a "plump" of ducks rose at the same time and took the route to the north in the wake of their noisier cousins / (Thoreau, 2004, pp. 301–302)

How many T-units are contained in this paragraph?   3

How many words did Thoreau use?   122

What is Thoreau's MLTU?   40.67

How many of Thoreau's T-units are complex sentences?   2

6. Upon the subject of education, not presuming to dictate any plan or system respecting it, I can only say that I view it as the most important subject which we as a people can be engaged in / that every man may receive at least a moderate education, and thereby be enabled to read the histories of his own and other countries, by which he may duly appreciate the value of our free institutions, appears to be an object of vital importance / (Abraham Lincoln, cited by Bachelder, 1965, p. 7)

How many T-units are contained in this paragraph?   2

How many words did Lincoln use?   81

What is Lincoln's MLTU?   40.50

How many of Lincoln's T-units are complex sentences?   2

7. I have been the whole day without eating and the whole night without sleeping, occupied with thinking / it was no use / the better plan is to learn / learning without thought is labor lost / and thought without learning is perilous / (Confucius, 6th century B.C., Peter Pauper Press, 1963, p. 42)

How many T-units are contained in this paragraph?   5

How many words did Confucius use?   39

What is Confucius's MLTU?   7.80

How many of Confucius's T-units are complex sentences?   4

8. The critical habit of thought, if usual in a society, will pervade all its mores, because it is a way of taking up the problems of life / men educated in it cannot be stampeded by stump orators and are never deceived by dithyrambic oratory / they are slow to believe / they can hold things as possible or probable in all degrees, without certainty and without pain / they can wait for evidence and weigh evidence, uninfluenced by the emphasis or confidence with which assertions are made on one side or the other / they can resist appeals to their dearest prejudices and all kinds of cajolery / education in the critical faculty is the only education of which it can be truly said that it makes good citizens / (William Graham Sumner, 1906, p. 633)

How many T-units are contained in this paragraph?   7

How many words did Sumner use?   124

What is Sumner's MLTU?   17.71

How many of Sumner's T-units are complex sentences?   5

9. Inside England, as we have seen, one form of the language, basically an East_Midland dialect, became accepted as a literary standard in the late Middle_Ages / and with this went a prestige accent based on that of the court in Westminster / this does not mean that dialect differences disappeared in England / Standard_English was the language of a small minority / most speakers used a nonstandard form of the language / and in each area there was a speech hierarchy corresponding to the class hierarchy, differing from Standard_English not only in accent but also in grammar and vocabulary / the higher the socioeconomic level of the speakers, the nearer their speech was likely to be to Standard_English, though the degree of formality of the situation also influenced the level of speech used / (Barber, 1993, p. 232)

How many T-units are contained in this paragraph?   7

How many words did Barber use?   127

What is Barber's MLTU?   18.14

How many of Barber's T-units are complex sentences?   5

10. We are a nation of Christians and Muslims, Jews, and Hindus, and non_believers / we are shaped by every language and culture, drawn from every end of this Earth / and because we have tasted the bitter swill of civil war and segregation, and emerged from that dark chapter stronger and more united, we cannot help but believe that the old hatreds shall someday pass, that the lines of tribe shall soon dissolve, that as the world grows smaller, our common humanity shall reveal itself, and that America must play its role in ushering in a new era of peace / (Barack Obama, 2009).

How many T-units are contained in this paragraph?   3

How many words did Obama use?   98

What is Obama's MLTU?   32.67

How many of Obama's T-units are complex sentences?   1

Exercise 13–2. Identifying Maze Behavior in Adolescent Speakers

The utterances here were produced by adolescents who were talking about sports and conflicts. For each utterance, use parentheses to enclose the maze behavior. What is left over should be a clean, coherent utterance, presumably the speaker's final formulation.

Speaker #1:

1. and (um you need to serve) when you serve, you need to serve behind the line, not over it.

2. (and then um in order to um in order to score over there you in or ok) when you serve and it goes over the net, and if the other players

do not hit it or if they can't get it and it's (in the) in the lines, then it's a point.

Speaker #2:

1. but usually the stadiums cost (maybe thirty or a lot of dollars) a lot of millions of dollars to put into it.

2. and they can play in any kind of weather (even) except for snow because they don't play in the snow.

3. and (a baseball game should last) a major league baseball game should last three hours.

Speaker #3:

1. (and and then there's) I don't know how many people play in pro.

2. but (I) we usually play five on five (like at school) like in sports for school.

3. and (um) that's about it.

Speaker #4:

1. and he asks (Peter if he would if) Mike to switch jobs with him because his (sh uh) shoulder was sore.

2. and he was like, "No, I don't wanna (lose) take a chance on losing my turn on the grill."

3. he could say, ("Okay but I get but one when one time when it's your time turn to be on the grill, you you need to let me) you cannot have a turn to use the grill when it's your turn, but this time I will do your garbage for you if you let me have it when you take your turn to use the grill."

Speaker #5:

1. he could say, "Bob (um you know) you were supposed to help us with this project and when you don't participate in the group, it frustrates me because it makes our group look bad and I'd appreciate it if you'd participate in the group."

2. (um he) unless Bob's an absolutely nasty person, he should get some kind of good results because he was pretty polite about it (and yeah).

Exercise 13–3. Calculating Clausal Density (CD)

Solve the following problems using the information that is provided.

1. 45 main clauses; 24 subordinate clauses; 45 C-units.   CD = 1.53

2. 82 main clauses; 68 subordinate clauses; 82 C-units.   CD = 1.83

3. 14 relative clauses; 20 adverbial clauses; 9 nominal clauses; 47 main clauses; 42 C-units.   CD = 2.14

4. 0 relative clauses; 17 adverbial clauses; 14 nominal clauses; 35 main clauses; 25 C-units utterances.   CD = 2.64

5. 15 relative clauses; 25 adverbial clauses; 16 nominal clauses; 60 main clauses; 60 C-units.   CD = 1.93

6. 10 adverbial clauses; 6 relative clauses; 9 nominal clauses; 4 infinitive clauses; 5 gerundive clauses; 5 participial clauses; 24 main clauses; 24 C-units.   CD = 2.63

7. 9 adverbial clauses; 0 relative clauses; 4 nominal clauses; 2 infinitive clauses; 0 gerundive clauses; 0 participial clauses; 16 main clauses; 16 C-units.   CD = 1.94

8. 4 adverbial clauses; 2 relative clauses; 2 nominal clauses; 4 infinitive clauses; 0 gerundive clauses; 0 participial clauses; 12 main clauses; 12 C-units.   CD = 2.0

CHAPTER 14: ANALYZING
LANGUAGE SAMPLES FROM ADOLESCENTS

Below are language samples (from the author's files) that were elicited from adolescents with typical language development. To elicit the samples, tasks were used that were described in Chapter 5 of this book. For each sample, indicate the types of main and subordinate clauses that occur, using the following codes: MC, ADV, REL, NOM, INF, PRT, GER.

E = examiner; C = adolescent

Sample #1: Conversation

Boy, Age 14 Years

MLCU = 9.93   CD = 1.70

E What would you like to tell me about yourself?

E For example, what could you tell me about school, or your family or friends or pets?

C (Um) at school I try **[MC]** to stay **[INF]** inclined.

C But I kind of get **[MC]** bored because I find **[ADV]** it somewhat boring.

C At home I try **[MC]** to do **[INF]** my chores.

C But I don't **[MC]** because (I don't really need any) I don't have **[ADV]** anything to do **[INF]** with the money after I get **[ADV]** it.

C And (um) I hang **[MC]** out with (a) a pretty tight group of friends.

E Are they all in cross-country?

C (Um) one of them is **[MC]**.

C And one of them is thinking **[MC]** about it.

C But they haven't really decided **[MC]** yet.

E How long have you been in cross-country?

C (Um) sixth grade.

E So two years.

E This is your second year?

C (Yes) no, this is [MC] my third.

C Started [MC] in sixth.

E Okay.

E And do you like it?

C (Um) It's [MC] a nice warmup for track, which I'm [REL] more into 'cause I'm [ADV] (kind of) better at track.

E Okay.

E What's your favorite track event?

C (Um) Pole vault.

E No way!

E Isn't that when you launch yourself over a tall pole?

C Yeah.

E You do that?

C (nods).

E Wow.

E Do you go to competitions for it?

C (Um) Well you're not allowed [MC] to do [INF] pole vault as a track event at other middle schools because I think [ADV] McArthur (is the only) has [NOM] the only (pole vault for like a) pole vault coach for middle school.

E So you can't compete with anyone.

C No.

E But you have a head start on competing.

C Yeah, I have **[MC]** a really big head start since I'm **[ADV]** (like) the best person in my grade right now.

C There's **[MC]** not really a lot of other people who do **[REL]** it, just two of my friends.

E What do you have to know to do pole vault well?

C (Um) You have **[MC]** to have **[INF]** good timing.

C (Uh) You have **[MC]** to be **[INF]** able to relax **[INF]** because if you (like) tighten **[ADV]** your abs when you're trying **[ADV]** to turn **[INF]** upside down to go **[INF]** over the pole, you'll **[ADV]** end up pulling **[GER]** on the bar and you might stretch **[ADV]** a muscle in your shoulder, which hurts **[REL]**.

C I've done **[MC]** that.

E You have?

E You stretched the muscle in your shoulder in pole vault?

C Yeah.

E Have you had any other track injuries?

C (Um well like) Yes, most of them are **[MC]** just (like) twisting **[GER]** ankles in long jump and stuff, though.

C They don't hurt **[MC]** as bad.

C It really hurts **[MC]**.

E How long does a twisted ankle take to recover?

C Like a day or two.

E Oh cool.

E But then you're back running full speed?

C I actually normally run **[MC]** with a twisted ankle.

C It kind of helps **[NOM]** stretch **[INF]** it out I think **[MC]**.

C But I try **[MC]** not to put **[INF]** a whole bunch of weight on it.

E That's really cool.

Sample #2: Conversation

Girl, Age 14 Years

MLCU = 9.41   CD = 1.59

E I am going to ask you a little bit about yourself.

C Well, I wish **[MC]** I worked **[NOM]**.

C But I don't **[MC]**.

C I have been trying **[MC]** to find **[INF]** a job this summer.

C But it appears **[MC]** no one is hiring **[NOM]** (um) inexperienced 14-year-olds.

C (Um) I baby sit **[MC]** for a kid named **[PRT]** Jacob.

C And he's **[MC]** really nice.

C He's **[MC]** ten and pretty mature.

C So it's **[MC]** kind of like being **[GER]** paid **[PRT]** (like) six dollars an hour to (um) play **[INF]** video games and watch **[INF]** TV with him and stuff.

C (Um my school) My school is **[MC]** Westminster_Middle_School.

C (Um it's uh) It's **[MC]** an okay school.

C I think **[MC]** that it's **[NOM]** a better fit for me than Southampton (but um it's).

E Why do you think that?

C (Uh) Well (we just) because (um) I was made **[MC]** fun of a lot when I was **[ADV]** in fifth and sixth grades.

C So at Southampton (I would have had) I feel **[MC]** like there is **[NOM]** just a more unfriendly atmosphere there.

C I'm **[MC]** not sure that I really like **[NOM]** the friends I have **[REL]** at my school (um).

C But I'm going **[MC]** into Woodbury_High_School.

C And (um) that's going **[MC]** to be **[INF]** a new experience for me (you know).

C Because I've never been **[MC]** to high school before.

C (Um) Actually, I'm **[MC]** quite familiar with one part of Woodbury_High_School.

C (I um) I am **[MC]** a theatre person.

C So (like um) I've been **[MC]** in a summer camp where they basically use **[ADV]** the entire (like) theatre and choir wing of Woodbury_High_School.

C And (I've been up) I've performed **[MC]** on that stage at least three times.

C (Um) I'm **[MC]** really into theatre and acting and stuff.

C In fact, (I was) my (uh) first professional role was **[MC]** in Sleeping_Beauty.

C (Um) It's **[MC]** the only professional role I've had **[REL]** yet because there's **[ADV]** just nothing up for kids although I am auditioning **[ADV]** for My_Fair_Lady.

C (Um uh) So we'll see **[MC]** how that goes **[NOM]**.

C (But um) I was **[MC]** in Sleeping_Beauty as a fairy.

C And (uh) over a hundred kids tried **[MC]** out.

C So I was **[MC]** pretty unprofessional.

C So I'm **[MC]** not quite sure how I got **[NOM]** in.

C But (uh) it was **[MC]** pretty fun.

C But so yeah.

C I performed **[MC]** on the community_center stage (um).

E When was that?

C That was **[MC]** when I was **[ADV]** in fifth grade.

C I think **[MC]** I was going **[NOM]** into fifth grade.

C Yeah, I was going **[MC]** into fifth grade.

C And (um) I was **[MC]** just a fairy (but).

E And did you speak?

C (Um) I sang **[MC]** on stage.

C But I didn't have **[MC]** any solos or anything.

C (Yeah I was) Yeah (uh) I ate **[MC]** like a mountain load of candy before every performance, which was **[REL]** not good for my voice I'm **[NOM]** sure (still but).

Sample #3: Conversation

Boy, Age 14 Years

MLCU = 7.76   CD = 1.18

E What would you like to tell me about yourself?

E For example, what could you tell me about school, or your family or friends or pets?

C (Well I have) My family is **[MC]** really close to me.

C Like (um) all my cousins and uncles and aunts live **[MC]** in Roseburg with me.

C And I see **[MC]** most of them almost every day.

C (Um).

E How many do you have?

C (I have) Both my grandma and grandpas live **[MC]** in Roseburg.

C I have **[NOM]** I think **[MC]** three aunts that live **[REL]** here and two uncles maybe.

E Do any of your aunts and uncles live elsewhere?

C (Uh) Yeah, actually I have **[MC]** an aunt and uncle in Bend.

C But I see **[MC]** them like five or six times a year.

E So you have a lot of cousins?

C Yeah, I have **[MC]** a lot of cousins.

E That sounds fun to me.

C (Um) Well (like) most of my family is **[MC]** (like) teachers or doctors.

C And then (my) one of my uncles that lives **[REL]** in Bend is **[MC]** an engineer.

E Oh cool.

C (Um) What else.

E Do you have pets?

C (Yeah I have) My sister has **[MC]** a turtle.

C And I have **[MC]** a dog.

E A turtle and a dog!

E Does the dog get along with the turtle?

C Well I guess **[MC]**.

C He doesn't try **[MC]** to bite **[INF]** him or anything.

E That's good.

E At least the turtle will be able to crawl into its shell.

E Does it live in a cage?

C Yeah, but (he like) sometimes my sister will let **[MC]** him out in the back yard to walk **[INF]** around in the summer.

E Is it big?

C Yeah, (it's like) well when we got **[ADV]** it, it was **[MC]** like that small.

C But now it's **[MC]** like that big.

E It's amazing how they grow!

C And it's **[MC]** supposed to be **[INF]** (like) like four feet by four feet when it gets **[ADV]** older.

C And they live **[MC]** like one hundred years.

E No way!

E How old is it now?

C (Um) Like three?

E Wow!

E It seems like it has grown a lot in three years.

C Uhhuh, yeah.

E So it will be really big, like one of those Galapagos Islands turtles.

E And so what is your dog like?

E What do you like to do with your dog?

C Well my dog is **[MC]** very small.

C He's **[MC]** a Chihuahua.

C He isn't **[MC]** really active.

C He just sits **[MC]** around all day.

E Is it a puppy or is it older?

C Well it's **[NOM]** like six I think **[MC]** now.

C But he is **[NOM]** I think **[MC]** a teacup Chihuahua.

C I'm [MC] not sure.

E Really!

E What's your favorite thing about him?

C (Um) I don't know [MC].

C Probably how (like) one second he can be [MC] like totally calm.

C But the other he will be [MC] very playful.

E He's unpredictable?

C And he listens [MC] pretty well.

E That's nice.

Sample #4: Mice in Council Narrative Retell

Boy, Age 14 Years

MLCU = 9.12   CD = 1.88

E Can you retell the story?

C (Uh) I could try [MC], yes.

C So (uh) these mice are living [MC] in fear of the cat.

C That ('s uh) happens [MC] a lot (I guess).

C And so (um) they decided [MC] to make [INF] a council because of the name of the story to try [INF] and figure [INF] out a way to (uh) solve [INF] this problem.

C Because (you know) they're losing [MC] a lot of people getting eaten [PRT] up by the cat.

C So they keep [MC] talking [GER] and talking [GER].

C And nothing seems [MC] to work [INF] (to work that would work).

C And one (mice) mouse was [MC] (uh) smart (I guess).

C (To uh) mice decided **[MC]** to (uh) make **[INF]** it so that the cat could be heard **[ADV]** by putting **[GER]** a bell around his neck.

C They thought **[MC]** it was **[NOM]** an amazing idea.

C So they applauded **[MC]**.

C And he gave **[MC]** a couple bows.

C And then (uh the) it was passed **[MC]** that they would do **[NOM]** this.

C 'Cause they have **[MC]** a little council.

C But (uh) then one old mouse that's **[REL]** wise (uh, uh) was (uh) congratulating **[MC]** him and thought **[MC]** of a question.

C (Uh) who would put **[MC]** the bell around the (mouse or) cat.

C And (uh) that's **[MC]** a good question.

E Awesome, nicely retold.

Sample #5: Mice in Council Narrative Retell

Girl, Age 14 Years

MLCU = 12.13   CD = 2.53

C (So) the mice were **[MC]** always in fear of this cat because (they'd always) he'd always approach **[ADV]** them and try **[ADV]** and eat **[INF]** them.

C And he'd toy **[MC]** with them and torture **[MC]** them.

C So the mice called **[MC]** together a council meeting.

C And they discussed **[MC]** many plans.

C But none of them seemed **[MC]** (to work or) like they were going **[NOM]** to work **[INF]**.

C And then a very small young mouse (um) approached **[MC]** and said **[MC]** that his idea was **[NOM]** to put **[INF]** a bell around the cat's neck so that whenever the cat came **[ADV]** they would hear **[ADV]** the bell tinkle **[INF]** and then they would know **[ADV]** he was coming **[NOM]** so they could escape **[ADV]**.

C And everyone thought **[MC]** it was **[NOM]** a really great idea.

C And so (um) they applauded **[MC]** him.

C And he took **[MC]** a few bows.

C And then (um) a wise older mouse stood **[MC]** up.

C And (said) this is **[MC]** basically what he said **[NOM]**.

C This is **[MC]** truly a great plan.

C And (um) only a genius could figure **[MC]** out a plan so simple (that we could) that we would have overlooked **[REL]**.

C And he says **[MC]** so now the question is **[NOM]** who's going **[NOM]** to put **[INF]** the bell on the cat.

C So basically things are **[MC]** easier said **[PRT]** than done **[PRT]**.

Sample #6: Monkey and Dolphin Narrative Retell

Boy, Age 14 Years

MLCU = 9.74   CD = 1.84

E Can you tell that story back to me?

C (Uh) so (uh) I guess **[MC]** it was **[NOM]** a custom to bring **[INF]** monkeys and other creatures along with them to amuse **[INF]** the (sailor) sailors.

C So one guy brought **[MC]** a monkey onto his boat.

C And they were sailing **[MC]** around somewhere (Uh) by (Greek) Greece (I guess).

C And (uh) there was **[MC]** a storm.

C The ship crashed **[MC]**.

C And everyone was **[MC]** in the water.

C And they were swimming **[MC]** towards shore.

C And so was **[MC]** the monkey.

C And then a dolphin, who must have **[REL]** bad eyesight to mistake **[INF]** a monkey for a man, (uh) swam **[MC]** up and grabbed **[MC]** the monkey with his back.

C And so the monkey had gotten **[MC]** onto him.

C And they're swimming **[MC]** there.

C And he asked **[MC]** him if he was **[NOM]** (a uh citizen) a Athenian.

C And the monkey said **[MC]** "yes" (you know) trying **[PRT]** to trick **[INF]** this dolphin because he's trying **[ADV]** to live **[INF]** on.

C And the dolphin asked **[MC]** him if he knew **[NOM]** something or someone.

C And the monkey, (you know) thinking **[PRT]** that oh yeah this must be **[NOM]** (uh) someone.

C Like oh yeah I know **[MC]** him.

C He's **[MC]** a dear friend.

C And the dolphin knew **[MC]** that he was lying **[NOM]**.

C So instead of saving **[GER]** him, he plunged **[MC]** down to the bottom to leave **[INF]** the monkey to his fate.

E Very nice.

Sample #7: Monkey and Dolphin Narrative Retell

Girl, Age 14 Years
MLCU = 13.29   CD = 2.21

C (Um) so it used **[MC]** to be **[INF]** (um) a custom that sailors would take **[REL]** on with them animals like a monkey or a dog to keep **[INF]** them entertained **[PRT]** on their long voyage.

C So on one particular (um) voyage, they took **[MC]** with them a monkey.

C And when they were **[ADV]** off the coast of Sunium, there was **[MC]** a terrible shipwreck.

C And everyone was turned **[MC]** overboard, including **[PRT]** the monkey.

C So a nearby dolphin (mis) mistook **[MC]** the monkey for a man.

C And so he came **[MC]** to his rescue.

C And then the dolphin asked **[MC]** him if he knew **[NOM]** Piraeus, which was **[REL]** also the name of the harbor off of Athens.

C And (um) he said **[MC]** yes I'm **[NOM]** (a) an Athenian.

C I'm **[MC]** from one of the first families that was **[REL]** here.

C And he said **[MC]** yes I knew **[NOM]** Piraeus.

C He's **[MC]** one of my oldest friends.

C And the dolphin knew **[MC]** then that he was (uh) not telling **[NOM]** the truth, that he was lying **[NOM]**.

C And so he dove **[MC]** deep into the water and left **[MC]** the monkey to his fate.

C And so the moral of the story would be **[MC]** people who pretend **[REL]** (uh) to be **[INF]** someone else basically end **[NOM]** up in deep water.

Sample #8: What Happened One Day, Narrative Essay

Boy, Age 17 Years

MLTU = 13.68   **CD = 2.58**

C One day a long time ago, my friend Jack and I went **[MC]** on a camping trip all by ourselves.

C We set **[MC]** up camp and went fishing **[MC]** to try **[INF]** and catch **[INF]** our dinner.

C I caught **[MC]** two fish while Jack caught **[ADV]** three.

C We were getting **[MC]** ready to leave **[INF]** when I looked **[ADV]** up the river and saw **[ADV]** this big dark blurry figure run **[INF]** off into the bushes.

C I didn't think **[MC]** anything of it.

C I just thought **[MC]** it was **[NOM]** an elk.

C On our way back to the camp, Jack started **[MC]** taunting **[GER]** me and bragging **[GER]** about how he was **[NOM]** a better fisherman than I was **[NOM]** because he caught **[ADV]** three fish while I only caught **[ADV]** two.

C We got **[MC]** back to camp.

C And I started **[MC]** a fire to cook **[INF]** the fish.

C I always started **[MC]** the fires.

C I was **[MC]** the best fire starter.

C We cooked **[MC]** some of our fish and put **[MC]** the rest in the ice chest for breakfast.

C We made **[MC]** our beds and went **[MC]** to sleep **[INF]**.

C Jack was still bragging **[MC]** about his fish.

C When I woke **[ADV]** in the morning, I opened **[MC]** my eyes to see **[INF]** Bigfoot eating **[PRT]** our fish.

C As I leaned **[ADV]** over to wake **[INF]** up Jack, it looked **[MC]** at me and ran **[MC]** off into the forest.

C Just like that, our camping trip turned **[MC]** into a hunt for rock solid proof of Bigfoot.

C After three days trying **[GER]** and failing **[GER]** to find **[INF]** Bigfoot anywhere, we gave **[MC]** up and went **[MC]** home.

C Ever since that day, I always have been **[MC]** sure to bring **[INF]** three things camping with me, a gun, a camera, and a better type of fishing bait.

Sample #9: Favorite Game or Sport Expository Task

Boy, Age 13 Years

MLTU = 10.16   CD = 1.67

E What is your favorite game or sport?

C My favorite sport in school would be **[MC]** wrestling.

E Why is wrestling your favorite sport?

C Well the (uh) coaches are **[MC]** really nice and everything.

C (we got got uh) We started **[MC]** out doing **[GER]** these (like uh) extra things.

C And (then uh and) then eventually I did **[MC]** everything and got **[MC]** good at it.

C So started **[MC]** getting **[GER]** gold medals and stuff.

E I'm not too familiar with the sport of wrestling, so I would like you to tell me all about it.

E For example, tell me what the goals are, and how many people may play a match.

E Also, tell me about the rules that players need to follow.

E Tell me everything you can think of about the sport of wrestling so that someone who has never played before would know how to play.

C (we) You start **[MC]** on a mat.

C You warm up **[MC]**.

C You go **[MC]** over to the mat.

C You shake **[MC]** hands.

C And the ref blows **[MC]** the whistle.

C And when you wrestle **[ADV]**, you start **[MC]** out neutral.

C And (you have to um you have to) you take **[MC]** the guy down by getting **[GER]** control of him while their hands or their feet are **[ADV]** on the mat.

C And if you're taking **[ADV]** a guy down (you can't like if you come around the back), you can't just pick **[MC]** them up and slap **[MC]** them on the mat.

C Otherwise it's **[MC]** unnecessary roughness.

C you get docked **[MC]** off a point.

C and if they are **[ADV]** (uh) too injured to wrestle **[INF]** then they win **[MC]** the match.

C and (um) it's **[MC]** really big on sportsmanship.

C so you can't go **[MC]** over and yell **[MC]** at the ref or yell **[MC]** at (the) them.

C Otherwise you'll get kicked **[MC]** for the next tournament.

C and (um yeah you also you have um you have to) you have **[MC]** to shake **[INF]** hands because it's **[ADV]** pretty much sportsmanship to do **[INF]** that.

C and once you get **[ADV]** the take down on them, you (um) try **[MC]** to break **[INF]** them down to their back.

C and you get **[MC]** them past a 45-degree angle.

C and you get **[MC]** near full points.

C then (uh) for 3 points, it's **[MC]** like 2 points.

C and (uh 5 points/s it/'s like 3 poin er uh) 5 seconds it's **[MC]** 3 points.

C and then after that, (you uh for how long) you hold **[MC]** them down.

C and it's **[MC]** about a 2-second pin.

C   and if you get **[ADV]** both their shoulders down and (uh them you uh) if you pin **[ADV]** them, you get **[MC]** to shake **[INF]** hands.

C   and you win **[MC]**.

C   but there's **[MC]** also points.

C   like for college, there's **[MC]** advantage time which is **[REL]** where (like somebody if) somebody was riding **[NOM]** a person for a long time.

C   and they get **[MC]** points.

C   (but once they go neutral then the timing down and stuff).

C   (so uh they have to kinda like) that's **[MC]** how it goes **[NOM]** with the advantage time.

C   They get **[MC]** certain amount of points at the end for advantage time and stuff.

C   (uh) it's **[MC]** pretty much big on sportsmanship.

C   and it's **[MC]** pretty easy to learn **[INF]**.

C   also you can't lock **[MC]** hands while they're **[ADV]** down around their waist (but) like around the leg (or around the ar).

C   but around the arm is **[MC]** okay.

C   (and stuff like that and can't like uh) in freestyle you can do **[MC]** that because it's **[ADV]** a big part of freestyle.

E   Now I would like you to tell me what a player should do in order to win the sport of wrestling.

E   In other words, what are some key strategies that every good player should know?

C   you just try **[MC]** to turn **[INF]** them so you get **[ADV]** back points.

C   and (uh once second) once both their shoulders touch **[ADV]** the mat, they're **[MC]** pinned.

E   Do they have to go all the way down?

C no you just have [MC] to get [INF] their shoulders to touch [INF].

E How long is a match?

C (um match/s are usually like in reg) I think [MC] they're [NOM] the same in everyone.

C so (they) for middle school, it's [MC] (like) about (like uh) three minutes or maybe four minutes or something like that.

C for high school it's [MC] six minutes.

C and college I'm [MC] not sure.

C I think [MC] it's [NOM] about the same as high school or (like) 30 seconds more or something.

E So a match isn't all that long.

C yeah it's [MC] not too hard (it's just) if you're [ADV] conditioned well and you have [ADV] a good work ethic.

C then you'll probably do [MC] well in wrestling.

C but if you don't try [ADV] your hardest, you're never going [MC] to get [INF] anywhere.

C yeah it's [MC] pretty much you can beat [NOM] guys that are [REL] strong as long as you have [ADV] a good technique.

C (but strength is kinda like) some people can just do [MC] bad technique and just knock [MC] you down and (um) then pin [MC] me and stuff.

C but most of the time you can get [MC] them.

E What about freestyle?

C (well in freestyle it's just you) I don't know [MC] much about freestyle.

C but you just touch [MC] (their both) their shoulders on the mat.

C and you win [MC].

C or you win **[MC]** by points at the end of the match.

C (same with collegiate except in collegiate it like 2 points pin).

C and (then like you'll uh and) if you don't pin **[ADV]** through the whole match, then you win **[MC]** by a certain amount of points.

C and then you get **[MC]** a certain amount of points for your team.

C but you can also technical **[MC]** them which is **[REL]** (like) when (you uh if) you (get) gain **[ADV]** (like) 15 points more than them.

C then they stop **[MC]** the match.

C and you win **[MC]**.

Sample #10: Peer Conflict Resolution Science Fair Task

Girl, Age 17 Years
MLCU = 15.40   **CD = 3.40**

E Now I'd like you to tell the story back to me, in your own words.

E Try to tell me everything you can remember about the story.

C The teacher gave **[MC]** the four girls an assignment to work **[INF]** together on a science project.

C And they decided **[MC]** they were going **[NOM]** to make **[INF]** a model airplane that could actually fly **[REL]**.

C And everyone worked **[MC]** on it except for one girl named **[PRT]** Melanie.

C And (it made Debbie angry or um) it made **[MC]** her indifferent because she wouldn't do **[ADV]** the work.

E What is the main problem here?

C (um) not everyone was participating **[MC]** equally or helping **[MC]** participating **[GER]**.

E Why is that a problem?

C Well if one person doesn't do **[ADV]** anything and they're **[ADV]** still in the group, they're still going **[MC]** to get **[INF]** the same grade.

C Or they're still going **[MC]** to be **[INF]** in that group as all the people that worked **[REL]** as hard.

C But they didn't contribute **[MC]** to it at all.

C So the other people may feel **[MC]** like they didn't deserve **[NOM]** it.

E What is a good way for Debbie to deal with Melanie?

C (um) I guess **[MC]** Debbie could ask **[NOM]** Melanie why she didn't want **[NOM]** to help **[INF]** or maybe she wanted **[NOM]** to do **[INF]** something different than what they wanted **[REL]** to do **[INF]**.

C Maybe that's **[MC]** the reason she didn't want **[REL]** to help **[INF]**.

C (or) And if that didn't work **[ADV]**, then she could ask **[MC]** the teacher to help **[INF]** them.

E Why is that a good way for Debbie to deal with Melanie?

C Because it's **[MC]** calm.

C She's not going **[MC]** to be **[INF]** like yelling **[PRT]** at her.

C They're going **[MC]** to try **[INF]** to compromise **[INF]** about it so that the three girls can do **[ADV]** what they want **[REL]** to do **[INF]**.

C But Melanie can also help **[MC]** since they're all contributing **[ADV]** to it.

E What do you think will happen if Debbie does that?

C (um) Maybe Melanie will say **[MC]** that she didn't want **[NOM]** to make **[INF]** an airplane or (she um) she wanted **[NOM]** to do **[INF]** something different.

C And so maybe they could interact **[MC]** that way and find **[MC]** out what the problem was **[NOM]** so Melanie could help **[ADV]** do **[INF]** something.

E How do you think they both will feel if Debbie does that?

C I think **[MC]** that they would kind of feel **[NOM]** more relaxed and not so uptight about her not helping **[GER]** or maybe Melanie not getting **[GER]** to do **[INF]** what she wants **[NOM]** to do **[INF]**.

C Maybe they would both feel **[MC]** more comfortable about the problem or talking **[GER]** about it.

Sample #11: Peer Conflict Resolution Fast Food Restaurant Task

Girl, Age 17 Years

MLCU = 11.63   CD = 2.21

E Now I'd like you to tell the story back to me, in your own words.

C (um Jane and Kathy) Jane is going **[MC]** to cook **[INF]** the food on the grill.

C And Kathy is going **[MC]** to take **[INF]** out the garbage.

C But her arm really hurts **[MC]**.

C And she wants **[MC]** to switch **[INF]** jobs.

C But Jane doesn't want **[MC]** to lose **[INF]** her spot at the grill.

E What is the main problem here?

C The main problem is **[MC]** that (maybe) maybe Jane doesn't want **[NOM]** to give **[INF]** up her spot.

C Maybe they could just switch **[MC]** for a minute for her to take **[INF]** out the garbage.

C Or maybe she could help **[MC]** Kathy take **[INF]** out the garbage.

C The main problem is **[MC]** that (they don't want to) Jane doesn't want **[NOM]** to switch **[INF]** jobs.

C But maybe she can just help **[MC]** Kathy instead do **[INF]** the grill.

E Why is that a problem?

C Because she said **[MC]** that she didn't want **[NOM]** to give **[INF]** up her spot at the grill.

C So obviously she didn't want **[MC]** to give **[INF]** up her spot at the grill.

C And (maybe) I don't know **[MC]** why.

E What is a good way for Jane to deal with Kathy?

C Well Jane could help **[MC]** Kathy take **[INF]** the garbage out.

C Or someone else could do **[MC]** it.

E Why is that a good way for Jane to deal with Kathy?

C Because they could both get **[MC]** their jobs done and help **[MC]** each other.

E What do you think will happen if Jane does that?

C I think **[MC]** that Kathy would really appreciate **[NOM]** it if Jane helped **[ADV]** her (and) and maybe in turn Kathy would help **[NOM]** Jane if she wanted **[ADV]** it.

C (or um) Then they could both get **[MC]** their jobs done.

E How do you think they both will feel if Jane does that?

C They'll both feel **[MC]** (like) happy that everything got done **[NOM]** or happy (that they solved) that they could help **[NOM]** each other and solve **[NOM]** the problems.

Sample #12: Nature of Friendship Expository Essay

Girl, Age 17 Years

MLTU = 12.48   **CD = 2.28**

C To me, friendship is **[MC]** a relationship between two or more people that like **[REL]** spending **[GER]** time with each other.

C A friend is **[MC]** someone you can talk **[REL]** to when there is **[ADV]** no other.

C You can tell **[MC]** them your secrets.

C And they will always have **[MC]** your back.

C If the world didn't have **[ADV]** friendship, then relationships and social status wouldn't mean **[MC]** a thing.

C The world would be **[MC]** full of people that don't like **[REL]** each other.

C And most of all, there wouldn't be **[MC]** anyone to talk **[INF]** with.

C Friends mostly keep **[MC]** you occupied.

C If I didn't have **[ADV]** friends, then my life would lack **[MC]** the excitement everyone needs **[REL]**.

C I would just wake **[MC]** up, go **[MC]** to school, come home **[MC]** and either watch **[MC]** TV or do **[MC]** nothing.

C With friends, it's **[MC]** like our lives are **[NOM]** all intertwined.

C And if one of us is doing **[ADV]** something exciting, then the rest should be **[MC]** in on it as well.

C Living **[GER]** a boring life isn't **[MC]** worth it.

C Usually friends share **[MC]** common interests.

C Either it being **[PRT]** culture, neighborhood, or personalities, they are **[MC]** usually like the other.

C Friendship to children is **[MC]** having **[GER]** someone to play **[INF]** with.

C Usually it's **[MC]** a person from school or a neighbor.

C For teenagers like me, friendship means **[MC]** someone to talk **[INF]** to when we get **[ADV]** in a fight with our parents, boyfriend, or girlfriends.

C Adults see **[MC]** friendship as more of a companionship.

C If they have **[ADV]** common interest in things, then they are **[MC]** more than likely to become **[INF]** friends.

C Or they have just been **[MC]** friends for a really long time.

C Usually people are **[MC]** friends one year then just are **[MC]** n't the next.

C People grow **[MC]** up and change **[MC]** and make **[MC]** new friends everyday.

C Sometimes friends just drift **[MC]** apart over the years.

C Other times, friends can do **[MC]** or say **[MC]** something that doesn't make **[REL]** them trustworthy.

C The usual result is **[MC]** a misunderstanding or someone gets **[NOM]** hurt.

C The best of friends are **[MC]** the ones that stay **[REL]** in touch for a really long time.

C There have been **[MC]** cases of people being **[GER]** friends since they were **[ADV]** three, and now at age sixty they are **[NOM]** still together.

C Friendships come **[MC]** and go **[MC]**, and depending **[PRT]** on what kind of friendship it is **[REL]**, can last **[MC]** a lifetime.

Sample #13: Circus Controversy Persuasive Essay

Boy, Age 17 Years

MLTU = 15.43   CD = 3.00

C Should animals perform **[MC]** in circuses?

C I believe **[MC]** that being **[GER]** trained to do **[INF]** tricks and to entertain **[INF]** audiences is **[NOM]** a very good use for animals.

C There are **[MC]**, however, a couple of sides on this subject.

C Some people think **[MC]** only of the entertainment with no concern for the animals' needs.

C Circuses may not feed **[MC]** the animals well or give **[MC]** them adequate space to live **[INF]** just for a little extra profit.

C It's **[MC]** also possible that they use **[NOM]** dangerous training techniques.

C These are **[MC]** all negative aspects on animals performing **[GER]** in circuses.

C There is **[MC]** also a good side to having **[GER]** circus animals.

C They can provide **[MC]** much entertainment for both adults and children, performing **[GER]** stunts, tricks, and acrobatics, jumping **[GER]** through fiery hoops, walking **[GER]** on hind legs, things you don't usually see **[REL]** your pets doing **[PRT]**.

C This can also help **[MC]** to eliminate **[INF]** any fears children might have **[REL]** of the performing animals.

C Looking **[PRT]** back at this reasoning and the impressions it gives **[REL]** us, I can see **[MC]** that there is **[NOM]** an easy solution to get **[INF]** rid of the negative aspects.

C Allow **[MC]** for the animals to perform **[INF]** in circuses, but only if they are **[ADV]** treated well, given **[ADV]** enough food, large enough living areas, and trained **[ADV]** without using **[GER]** too harsh punishment.

C Using **[PRT]** this method, there are **[MC]** only positive reasons.

C So why not have **[MC]** animals perform **[INF]** in circuses?

Sample #14: Circus Controversy Persuasive Essay

Girl, Age 18 Years
MLTU = 11.69   CD = 2.38

C I feel **[MC]** that animals performing **[GER]** for our entertainment is **[NOM]** a bad idea!

C We have **[MC]** many other forms of entertainment in this day and age.

C We do not need **[MC]** to force **[INF]** wild animals to do **[INF]** things for our entertainment.

C The animals that are **[REL]** part of circuses do not have **[MC]** the proper habitat that they need **[REL]**.

C They do not have **[MC]** space that they need **[REL]**.

C And they have been known **[MC]** to become **[INF]** violent.

C I do not have **[MC]** a problem with people performing **[GER]**, with cats and dogs, even horses.

C But all of these are **[MC]** domestic animals.

C Tigers, bears, and elephants should not be **[MC]** locked **[PRT]** in small cages, forced **[PRT]** to do **[INF]** tricks, and be **[MC]** poorly treated **[PRT]**.

C There is **[MC]** no reason that people and domestic animals could not give **[REL]** just as good of a performance.

C Wild animals are **[MC]** just that, wild.

C They need **[MC]** to be **[INF]** in habitats that are **[REL]** suitable for them.

C They need **[MC]** to be **[INF]** fed **[PRT]** right and let **[PRT]** to use **[INF]** their instincts.

C Malnutrition, small confined areas, and entertainment for people is **[MC]** not what these creatures are **[REL]** on this earth for.

C They are **[MC]** animals, not actors.

C And we need **[MC]** to remember **[INF]** this.

References

Afflerbach, P., Beers, J. W., Blachowicz, C., Boyd, C. D., & Diffily, D. (2000). *Scott Foresman reading: Fantastic Voyage* (Vols. 1 & 2). Glenview, IL: Scott Foresman.

Bachelder, L. (1965). *Abraham Lincoln: Wisdom and wit*. Mount Vernon, NY: Peter Pauper Press.

Bamberg, M. (1994). Development of linguistic forms: German. In R. A. Berman & D. I. Slobin (Eds.), *Relating events in narrative: A cross-linguistic developmental study* (pp. 189–238). Hillsdale, NJ: Erlbaum.

Bamberg, M., & Damrad-Frye, R. (1991). On the ability to provide evaluative comments: Further explorations of children's narrative competencies. *Journal of Child Language, 18*, 689–710.

Bannister, R. (2004). *The four-minute mile: 50th anniversary edition*. Guilford, CT: Lyons Press.

Barber, C. (1993). *The English language: A historical introduction*. Cambridge, UK: Cambridge University Press.

Baron-Cohen, S., Wheelwright, S., Lawson, J., Griffin, R., Ashwin, C., Billington, J., & Chakrabarti, B. (2005). Empathizing and systemizing in autism spectrum conditions. In F. R. Volkmar, R. Paul, A. Klin, & D. Cohen (Eds.), *Handbook of autism and pervasive developmental disorders, Volume 1: Diagnosis, development, neurobiology, and behavior* (3rd ed., pp. 628–639). Hoboken, NJ: John Wiley.

Bearison, D. J., & Gass, S. T. (1979). Hypothetical and practical reasoning: Children's persuasive appeals in different social contexts. *Child Development, 50*, 901–903.

Behrens, H. (2008). Corpora in language acquisition research: History, methods, perspectives. In H. Behrens (Ed.), *Corpora in language acquisition research: History, methods, perspectives* (pp. xi–xxx). Philadelphia, PA: John Benjamins.

Benardete, D. (1961). *Mark Twain: Wit and wisecracks*. Mount Vernon, NY: Peter Pauper Press.

Bennett, T., Szatmari, P., Bryson, S., Volden, J., Zwaigenbaum, L., Vaccarella, L., Duku, E., & Boyle, M. (2008). Differentiating autism and Asperger syndrome on the basis of language delay or impairment. *Journal of Autism and Developmental Disorders, 38*, 616–625.

Berman, R. (Ed.). (2004). *Language development across childhood and adolescence*. Amsterdam, The Netherlands: John Benjamins.

Berman, R. (2008). The psycholinguistics of developing text construction. *Journal of Child Language, 35*(4), 735–771.

Berman, R., & Nir, B. (2010). The language of expository discourse across adolescence. In M. A. Nippold & C. M. Scott (Eds.), *Expository discourse in children, adolescents, and adults: Development and disorders* (pp. 99–121). New York, NY: Psychology Press/Taylor & Francis.

Berman, R. A., & Slobin, D. I. (Eds.). (1994). *Relating events in narrative: A crosslinguistic developmental study*. Hillsdale, NJ: Lawrence Erlbaum Associates.

Berman, R. A., & Verhoeven, L. (2002). Cross-linguistic perspectives on the development of text-production abilities: Speech and writing. *Written Language and Literacy, 5*(1), 1–43.

Berry, M. F. (1969). *Language disorders of children: The bases and diagnoses*. Englewood Cliffs, NJ: Prentice-Hall.

Biggs, A., Gregg, K., Hagins, W. C., Kapicka, C., Lundgren, L., Rillero, P., & National Geographic Society. (2002). *Biology: The dynamics of life*. New York, NY: Glencoe/McGraw-Hill.

Bishop, D. V. M. (2004). *Expression, reception, and recall of narrative instrument (ERRNI)*. London, UK: Harcourt Assessment.

Bishop, D. V. M., & Donlan, C. (2005). The role of syntax in encoding and recall of pictorial narratives: Evidence from specific language impairments. *British Journal of Developmental Psychology, 23*, 25–46.

Bloom, L. (1970). *Language development: Form and function in emerging grammars*. Cambridge, MA: MIT Press.

Bloom, L., & Lahey, M. (1978). *Language development and language disorders*. New York, NY: John Wiley & Sons.

Botvin, G. J., & Sutton-Smith, B. (1977). The development of structural complexity in children's fantasy narratives. *Developmental Psychology, 13*, 377–388.

Bragg, B. W. E., Ostrowski, M. V., & Finley, G. E. (1973). The effects of birth order and age of target on use of persuasive techniques. *Child Development, 44*, 351–354.

Braine, M. (1963). The ontogeny of English phrase structure: The first phrase. *Language, 39*, 1–13.

Brinton, B., Robinson, L. A., & Fujiki, M. (2004). Description of a program for social language intervention: "If you can have a conversation, you can have a relationship." *Language, Speech, and Hearing Services in Schools, 35*, 283–290.

Brown, R. (1973). *A first language: The early stages*. Cambridge, MA: Harvard University Press.

Burke, N. (1996). *Teachers are special: A tribute to those who educate, encourage, and inspire*. New York, NY: Gramercy Books.

Category: Proverbs. (2009). Retrieved from http://www.en.wiki quote.org/wiki/

Chaisson, E., & McMillan, S. (2005). *Astronomy today* (5th ed.). Upper Saddle River, NJ: Pearson Prentice Hall.

Charlton, J. (Ed.). (1994). *A little learning is a dangerous thing*. New York, NY: St. Martins Press.

Chomsky, N. (1957). *Syntactic structures*. The Hague, Netherlands: Mouton.

Chomsky, N. (1965). *Aspects of the theory of syntax*. Cambridge, MA: MIT Press.

Clark, R. A., & Delia, J. G. (1976). The development of functional persuasive skills in childhood and early adolescence. *Child Development, 47,* 1008–1014.

Creative proverbs from around the world. (2009). Retrieved from http://www.creativeproverbs.com/

Crews, F. (1977). *The Random House handbook* (2nd ed.). New York, NY: Random House.

Crowhurst, M. (1980). Syntactic complexity in narration and argument at three grade levels. *Canadian Journal of Education, 5,* 6–13.

Crowhurst, M. (1987). Cohesion in argument and narration at three grade levels. *Research in the Teaching of English, 21,* 185–201.

Crowhurst, M. (1990). Teaching and learning the writing of persuasive/argumentative discourse. *Canadian Journal of Education, 15,* 348–359.

Crowhurst, M., & Piche, G. L. (1979). Audience and mode of discourse effects on syntactic complexity in writing at two grade levels. *Research in the Teaching of English, 13,* 101–109.

Crystal, D. (1996). *Rediscover grammar with David Crystal* (Rev. ed.). Essex, UK: Longman.

Crystal, D. (2002). *The English language: A guided tour of the language* (2nd ed.). London, UK: Penguin Books.

Crystal, D., Fletcher, P., & Garman, M. (1976). *The grammatical analysis of language disability.* London, UK: Edward Arnold.

Darwin, C. (1877). A biographical sketch of an infant. *Mind, 2,* 285–294.

Darwin, C. (1958). In N. Barlow (Ed.), *The autobiography of Charles Darwin (1809–1882).* New York, NY: Norton & Company.

Davies, H. (1989). *The good guide to the lakes* (3rd ed.). Loweswater, UK: Forster Davies.

Delia, J. G., Kline, S. L., & Burleson, B. R. (1979). The development of persuasive communication strategies in kindergarten through twelfth-graders. *Communication Monographs, 46,* 241–256.

de Villiers, J. G., & de Villiers, P. A. (1973). A cross-sectional study of the acquisition of grammatical morphemes. *Journal of Psycholinguistic Research, 2,* 267–278.

Dumond, V. (1993). *Grammar for grownups.* New York, NY: HarperCollins.

Eder, D. (1988). Building cohesion through collaborative narration. *Social Psychology Quarterly, 51,* 225–235.

Eisenberg, S. L. (2006). Grammar: How can I say that better? In T. A. Ukrainetz (Ed.), *Contextualized language intervention: Scaffolding PreK–12 literacy achievement* (pp. 145–194). Eau Claire, WI: Thinking Publications.

Emerson, R. W. (2009/1841). Self-reliance. In Penguin Books (Ed.), *Barack Obama: The inaugural address together with Abraham Lincoln's first and second inaugural addresses and the Gettysburg Address and Ralph Waldo Emerson's Self-Reliance.* New York, NY: Penguin Books.

Epstein, S., & Phillips, J. (2009). Storytelling skills of children with specific language impairment. *Child Language Teaching and Therapy, 25*(3), 285–300.

Erftmier, T., & Dyson, A. H. (1986). "Oh ppbbt!": Differences between the oral and written persuasive strategies of school-aged children. *Discourse Processes, 9,* 91–114.

Fanning, J. L. (2004, November). *Persuasive writing abilities in school-age children, adolescents, and adults: Applying the data.* Seminar presented at the

Annual Convention of the American Speech-Language-Hearing Association, Philadelphia, PA.

Felton, M., & Kuhn, D. (2001). The development of argumentative discourse skill. *Discourse Processes, 32*(2/3), 135–153.

Feynman, R. P. (1996). Introduction to computers. In A. J. G. Hey & R. W. Allen (Eds.), *Feynman lectures on computation* (pp. 1–19). Reading, MA: Addison-Wesley.

Finley, G. E., & Humphreys, C. A. (1974). Naïve psychology and the development of persuasive appeals in girls. *Canadian Journal of Behavioral Science, 6*, 75–80.

Flavell, J. H., Botkin, P. T., Fry, C. L., Wright, J. W., & Jarvis, P. E. (1968). *The development of role-taking and communication skills in children*. New York, NY: Wiley.

Fuller, M. (1999/1845). In J. T. Pine (Ed.), *Woman in the nineteenth century. Dover Thrift Editions*. New York, NY: Dover.

Gage, J. T. (1991). *The shape of reason: Argumentative writing in college* (2nd ed.). New York, NY: Macmillan.

Geurts, H. M., & Embrechts, M. (2008). Language profiles in ASD, SLI, and ADHD. *Journal of Autism and Developmental Disorders, 38*, 1931–1943.

Gillam, R. B., & Pearson, N. A. (2004). *Test of Narrative Language (TNL)*. East Moline, IL: LinguiSystems.

Graham, S., & Perin, D. (2007). A meta-analysis of writing instruction for adolescent students. *Journal of Educational Psychology, 99*(1), 445–476.

Grammar: Parts of speech. (2009). Retrieved from http://www.eslus.com/LESSONS/GRAMMAR/POS/pos1.htm

Great Quotations. (1990). *Teacher's inspirations: Motivational quotes for you and your students*. Glendale Heights, IL: Great Quotations.

Grosset & Dunlap. (1947). *Aesop's fables*. New York, NY: Author.

Hadley, P. A. (1998). Language sampling protocols for eliciting text-level discourse. *Language, Speech, and Hearing Services in Schools, 29*, 132–147.

Ham, A., Burke, A., Carillet, J., Kohn, M., Gordon, F. L., Maxwell, V., & Mayhew, B. (2006). *Middle East* (5th ed.). Oakland, CA: Lonely Planet.

Harris, J. (1989). *The land and people of France*. New York, NY: Lippincott.

Hauser, S. (2008). *The proverbial cat: 2009 calendar*. Portland, ME: Sellers.

Hirschman, M. (2000). Language repair via metalinguistic means. *International Journal of Language and Communication Disorders, 35*(2), 252–268.

Hoskins, B. (1996). *Conversations: A framework for language intervention* (Rev. ed.). Eau Claire, WI: Thinking Publications.

Howlin, P. (2005). Outcomes in autism spectrum disorders. In F. R. Volkmar, R. Paul, A. Klin, & D. Cohen (Eds.), *Handbook of autism and pervasive developmental disorders, Volume 1: Diagnosis, development, neurobiology, and behavior* (3rd ed., pp. 201–221). Hoboken, NJ: John Wiley.

Humphreys, M. W. (1880). A contribution to infantile linguistics. *Transactions of the American Philological Association, 11*, 5–17.

Hunt, K. W. (1970). Syntactic maturity in school children and adults. *Monographs of the Society for Research in Child Development*, Serial No. 134, Volume 35, No. 1.

Ingram, D. (1989). *First language acquisition: Method, description, and explanation*. Cambridge, UK: Cambridge University Press.

Jarvie, G. (2007). *Bloomsbury grammar guide* (2nd ed.). London, UK: A & C Black.

Jones, D. C. (1985). Persuasive appeals and responses to appeals among friends and acquaintances. *Child Development, 56*, 757–763.

Jones, R. M., McLeod, J. C., Krockover, G. H, Frank, M. S., Lang, M. P., Valenta, C. J., & Van Deman, B. A. (2002). *Harcourt science teacher's edition, life science units A and B*. Orlando, FL: Harcourt.

Justice, L. M., Bowles, R. P., Kaderavek, J. N., Ukrainetz, T. A., Eisenberg, S. L., & Gillam, R. B. (2006). The index of narrative microstructure: A clinical tool for analyzing school-age children's narrative performances. *American Journal of Speech-Language Pathology, 15*, 177–191.

Kernan, K. T. (1977). Semantic and expressive elaboration in children's narratives. In S. Ervin-Tripp & C. Mitchell-Kernan (Eds.), *Child discourse* (pp. 91–102). New York, NY: Academic Press.

Klecan-Aker, J. S., & Caraway, T. H. (1997). A study of the relationship of storytelling ability and reading comprehension in fourth and sixth grade African-American children. *European Journal of Disorders of Communication, 32*, 109–125.

Knudson, R. E. (1992). The development of written argumentation: An analysis and comparison of argumentative writing at four grade levels. *Child Study Journal, 22*, 167–184.

Kroll, B. M. (1984). Audience adaptation in children's persuasive letters. *Written Communication, 1*, 407–427.

Landa, R. J., & Goldberg, M. C. (2005). Language, social, and executive functions in high functioning autism: A continuum of performance. *Journal of Autism and Developmental Disorders, 35*, 557–573.

Larson, V. L., & McKinley, N. (2003). *Communication solutions for older students: Assessment and intervention strategies*. Eau Claire, WI: Thinking Publications.

Launer, P. B., & Lahey, M. (1981). Passages: From the fifties to the eighties in language assessment. *Topics in Language Disorders, 1*(3), 11–29.

Lawrence, J. (1997). *Aesop's Fables*. Seattle, WA: University of Washington Press.

Leadholm, B. J., & Miller, J. F. (1992). *Language sample analysis: The Wisconsin guide*. Madison, WI: Wisconsin Department of Public Instruction.

Lee, L. L. (1974). *Developmental sentence analysis: A grammatical assessment procedure for speech and language clinicians*. Evanston, IL: Northwestern University Press.

Lee, L. L., & Canter, S. M. (1971). Developmental sentence scoring: A clinical procedure for estimating syntactic development in children's spontaneous speech. *Journal of Speech and Hearing Disorders, 36*, 315–340.

Leopold, W. F. (1939–1949). *Speech development of a bilingual child: A linguist's record* (Vols. 1–4). Evanston, IL: Northwestern University Press.

Lewis, F. M., Murdoch, B. E., & Woodyatt, G. C. (2007). Communicative competence and metalinguistic ability: Performance by children and adults with autism spectrum disorder. *Journal of Autism and Developmental Disorders, 37*, 1525–1538.

Liles, B. Z. (1985). Narrative ability in normal and language disordered children. *Journal of Speech and Hearing Research, 28*, 123–133.

Liles, B. Z. (1987). Episode organization and cohesive conjunctives in narratives of children with and without language disorders. *Journal of Speech and Hearing Research, 30*, 185–196.

Liles, B. Z. (1993). Narrative discourse in children with language disorders and children with normal language: A critical review of the literature. *Journal of Speech and Hearing Research, 36*, 868–882.

Liles, B. Z., Duffy, R. J., Merritt, D. D., & Purcell, S. L. (1995). Measurement of narrative discourse ability in children with language disorders. *Journal of Speech and Hearing Research, 38,* 415–425.

Loban, W. (1976). *Language development: Kindergarten through grade twelve.* Urbana, IL: National Council of Teachers of English.

Long, S., & Fey, M. (1993). *Computerized profiling* [Computer program; version 7.2]. Ithaca, NY: Computerized Profiling.

Loveland, K. A., & Tunali-Kotoski, B. (2005). The school-age child with an autistic spectrum disorder. In F. R. Volkmar, R. Paul, A. Klin, & D. Cohen (Eds.), *Handbook of autism and pervasive developmental disorders, Volume 1: Diagnosis, development, neurobiology, and behavior* (3rd ed., pp. 247–287). Hoboken, NJ: John Wiley.

Luciano, A., Batzella, G., Borghese, D. A. S., Borghese, D. M., Callen, A. T., Carluccio, A., . . . Rando, R. (1991). *Italy: A culinary journey.* San Francisco, CA: Collins.

Lynch, J. (1978). Evaluation of linguistic disorders in children. In S. Singh & J. Lynch, *Diagnostic procedures in hearing, language, and speech* (pp. 327–378). Baltimore, MD: University Park Press.

MacWhinney, B. (1988). *CLAN: Child Language Analysis: Manual for the CLAN programs of the Child Language Data Exchange System.* Pittsburgh, PA: Carnegie Mellon University.

Marinellie, S. A. (2004). Complex syntax used by school-age children with specific language impairment (SLI) in child-adult conversation. *Journal of Communication Disorders, 37,* 517–533.

Mayer, M. (1969). *Frog where are you?* New York, NY: Dial Press.

McCabe, A., Bliss, L., Barra, G., & Bennett, M. (2008). Comparison of personal versus fictional narratives of children with language impairment. *American Journal of Speech-Language Pathology, 17,* 194–206.

McCann, T. M. (1989). Student argumentative writing knowledge and ability at three grade levels. *Research in the Teaching of English, 23,* 62–76.

McCarthy, D. (1930). The language development of the preschool child. *Institute of Child Welfare Monograph Series 4.* Minneapolis, MN: University of Minnesota Press.

McClenaghan, W. A. (2005). *Magruder's American government* (Teacher's ed.). Upper Saddle River, NJ: Pearson Prentice Hall.

McDougal Littell. (2006). *The language of literature: British literature* (Teacher's ed.). Evanston, IL: McDougal Littell/Houghton Mifflin.

McLellan, V. (1996). *The complete book of practical proverbs and wacky wit.* Wheaton, IL: Tyndale House.

Merritt, D. D., & Liles, B. Z. (1987). Story grammar ability in children with and without language disorders: Story generation, story retelling, and story comprehension. *Journal of Speech and Hearing Research, 30,* 539–551.

Merritt, D. D., & Liles, B. Z. (1989). Narrative analysis: Clinical applications of story generation and story retelling. *Journal of Speech and Hearing Disorders, 54,* 438–447.

Microsoft Word. (2007). *Flesch-Kincaid Grade Level Readability.* Redmond, WA: Microsoft Corporation.

Miller, J. F. (1981). *Assessing language production in children: Experimental procedures.* Baltimore, MD: University Park Press.

Miller, J. F. (2009). New database: Helps identify, monitor older students. *Advance for Speech-Language Pathologists & Audiologists, 19*(8), 4–7.

Miller, J. F., & Chapman, R. (1983). *Systematic analysis of language transcripts.* Madison, WI: University of Wisconsin-Madison, Language Analysis Laboratory, Waisman Center on Mental Retardation and Human Development.

Miller, J. F., & Chapman, R. (2003). *SALT: Systematic Analysis of Language Transcripts* [Computer software]. Madison, WI: University of Wisconsin-Madison, Waisman Center, Language Analysis Laboratory.

Miller, W., & Ervin, S. (1964). The development of grammar in child language. In U. Bellugi & R. Brown (Eds.), *The acquisition of language: Monograph of the Society for Research in Child Development, 29,* Serial No. 92, 9–34.

Moffet, C. (2006). Sarkis Antikajian. *Jerry Williams' Quarterly, 3*(3), 18–19.

Moran, C., & Gillon, G. T. (2010). Expository discourse in older children and adolescents with traumatic brain injury. In M. A. Nippold & C. M. Scott (Eds.), *Expository discourse in children, adolescents, and adults: Development and disorders* (pp. 275–301). New York, NY: Psychology Press/Taylor & Francis.

Moran, C., Kirk, C., & Powell, E. (2012). Spoken persuasive discourse abilities of adolescents with acquired brain injury. *Language, Speech, and Hearing Services in Schools, 43,* 264–275.

National Governors Association Center for Best Practices and Council of Chief State School Officers. (2010). *Common core state standards for English language arts.* Retrieved from http://www.corestandards.org

Nelson, N. W. (1998). *Childhood language disorders in context: Infancy through adolescence* (2nd ed.). Boston, MA: Allyn & Bacon.

Nelson, N. W. (2010). *Language and literacy disorders: Infancy through adolescence.* Boston, MA: Allyn & Bacon.

Nippold, M. A. (1999). Word definition in adolescents as a function of reading proficiency. *Child Language Teaching and Therapy, 15*(2), 171–176.

Nippold, M. A. (2000). Language development during the adolescent years: Aspects of pragmatics, syntax, and semantics. *Topics in Language Disorders, 20*(2), 15–28.

Nippold, M. A. (2007). *Later language development: School-age children, adolescents, and young adults* (3rd ed.). Austin, TX: Pro-Ed.

Nippold, M. A. (2009). School-age children talk about chess: Does knowledge drive syntactic complexity? *Journal of Speech, Language, and Hearing Research, 52,* 856–871.

Nippold, M. A. (2010a). Explaining complex matters: How knowledge of a domain drives language. In M. A. Nippold & C. M. Scott (Eds.), *Expository discourse in children, adolescents, and adults: Development and disorders* (pp. 41–61). New York, NY: Psychology Press/Taylor & Francis.

Nippold, M. A. (2010b). It's NOT too late to help adolescents succeed in school [From the editor]. *Language, Speech, and Hearing Services in Schools, 41,* 137–138.

Nippold, M. A., Cramond, P. M., & Hayward-Mayhew, C. (2014). Spoken language production in adults: Examining age-related differences in syntactic complexity. *Clinical Linguistics & Phonetics.* Advance online publication.

Nippold, M. A., Frantz-Kaspar, M. W., Cramond, P., Kirk, C., Hayward-Mayhew, C., & MacKinnon, M. (2014). Conversational and narrative speaking in adolescents: Examining the use of complex syntax. *Journal of Speech, Language, and Hearing Research.* Advance online publication. doi:10.1044/1092-4388

Nippold, M. A., Hegel, S. L., Sohlberg, M. M., & Schwarz, I. E. (1999). Defining abstract entities: Development in pre-adolescents, adolescents, and young adults. *Journal of Speech, Language, and Hearing Research, 41*(2), 473–481.

Nippold, M. A., & Hesketh, L. J. (2009, June). *Expository discourse in adolescents with autism spectrum disorders: Examining the use of complex syntax.* Poster presented at the 30th Anniversary of the Symposium on Research in Child Language Disorders, University of Wisconsin, Madison, WI.

Nippold, M. A., Hesketh, L. J., Duthie, J. K., & Mansfield, T. C. (2005). Conversational versus expository discourse: A study of syntactic development in children, adolescents, and adults. *Journal of Speech, Language, and Hearing Research, 48*, 1048–1064.

Nippold, M. A., Mansfield, T. C., & Billow, J. L. (2007). Peer conflict explanations in children, adolescents, and adults: Examining the development of complex syntax. *American Journal of Speech-Language Pathology, 16*, 179–188.

Nippold, M. A., Mansfield, T. C., Billow, J. L., & Tomblin, J. B. (2008). Expository discourse in adolescents with language impairments: Examining syntactic development. *American Journal of Speech-Language Pathology, 17*, 356–366.

Nippold, M. A., Mansfield, T. C., Billow, J. L., & Tomblin, J. B. (2009). Syntactic development in adolescents with a history of language impairments: A follow-up investigation. *American Journal of Speech-Language Pathology, 18*, 241–251.

Nippold, M. A., Moran, C., Mansfield, T. C., & Gillon, G. (2005, July). *Expository discourse development in American and New Zealand youth: A cross-cultural comparison.* Poster presented at the Xth International Congress for the Study of Child Language (IASCL), Freie Universitat, Berlin, Germany.

Nippold, M. A., & Scott, C. M. (2010). Overview of expository discourse: Development and disorders. In M. A. Nippold & C. M. Scott (Eds.), *Expository discourse in children, adolescents, and adults: Development and disorders* (pp. 1–11). New York, NY: Psychology Press/Taylor & Francis.

Nippold, M. A., & Sun, L. (2010). Expository writing in children and adolescents: A classroom assessment tool. *Perspectives on Language Learning and Education: Adolescent Language, 17*, 100–107. Published by Division 1, American Speech-Language-Hearing Association.

Nippold, M. A., & Ward-Lonergan, J. (2010). Argumentative writing in preadolescents: The role of verbal reasoning. *Child Language Teaching and Therapy, 26*, 238–248.

Nippold, M. A., Ward-Lonergan, J., & Fanning, J. L. (2005). Persuasive writing in children, adolescents, and adults: A study of syntactic, semantic, and pragmatic development. *Language, Speech, and Hearing Services in Schools, 36*, 125–138.

Obama, B. (2009). *Inaugural address.* New York, NY: Penguin Books.

Oliva-Rasbach, J., & Schmidt, C. W. (1994). *Viva la Mediterranean.* Englewood, CO: HealthMark Centers.

Parker, J. L. (2009). *Once a runner: A novel* (1st Scribner hardcover ed.). New York, NY: Scribner/Simon & Schuster.

Paul, R. (2007). *Language disorders from infancy through adolescence: Assessment and intervention* (3rd ed.). St Louis, MO: Mosby/Elsevier.

Paul, R., & Norbury, C. F. (2012). *Language disorders from infancy through adolescence: Listening, speaking, read, writing, and communicating* (4th ed.). St. Louis, MO: Elsevier.

Paul, R., Orlovski, S. M., Marcinko, H. C., & Volkmar, F. (2009). Conversational behaviors in youth with high-functioning ASD and Asperger syndrome. *Journal of Autism and Developmental Disorders, 39*, 115–125.

Peter Pauper Press. (1963). *The wisdom of Confucius.* Mount Vernon, NY: Peter Pauper Press.

Piche, G. L., Rubin, D. L., & Michlin, M. L. (1978). Age and social class in children's use of persuasive communicative appeals. *Child Development, 49*, 773–780.

Politis, V., Reich, A. A., & Sheldon, R. (1998). *Russian proverbs: 100 favorites of Professor Nadezhda Timofeevna Koroton.* Hanover, NH: Dartmouth Triad Associates.

Popham, P. (1992). *The insider's guide to Japan.* Edison, NJ: Hunter.

Preyer, W. (1889). *The mind of the child* (Translation of the original German edition of 1882). New York, NY: Appleton.

Quirk, R., & Greenbaum, S. (1973). *A concise grammar of contemporary English.* New York, NY: Harcourt Brace Jovanovich.

Quotable Shakespeare. (n.d.). *A knowledge cards deck from the plays of William Shakespeare.* Rohnert Park, CA: Pomegranate.

Quotations Page. Retrieved from www.quotationspage.com

Retherford, K. (1993). *Guide to analysis of language transcripts* (2nd ed.). Eau Claire, WI: Thinking Publications.

Reutzel, D. R. (2009). Reading fluency: What every SLP and teacher should know. *ASHA Leader, 14*(5), 10, 12–13.

Ritter, E. M. (1979). Social perspective-taking ability, cognitive complexity, and listener-adapted communication in early and late adolescence. *Communication Monographs, 46*, 40–51.

Robertson, S. (2009). Connecting reading fluency and oral language for student success. *ASHA Leader, 14*(5), 11.

Robinson, D., & Groves, J. (2004). *Introducing philosophy.* Thriplow, Cambridge, UK: Icon Books.

Robinson, D., & Groves, J. (2005). *Introducing Plato.* Thriplow, Cambridge, UK: Icon Books.

Roth, F. P., & Spekman, N. J. (1986). Narrative discourse: Spontaneously generated stories of learning-disabled and normally achieving students. *Journal of Speech and Hearing Disorders, 51*, 8–23.

Rubin, D. L., & Piche, G. L. (1979). Development in syntactic and strategic aspects of audience adaptation skills in written persuasive communication. *Research in the Teaching of English, 13*, 293–316.

Saddler, B., & Graham, S. (2005). The effects of peer-assisted sentence-combining instruction on the writing performance of more and less skilled young writers. *Journal of Educational Psychology, 97*(1), 43–54.

Santrock, J. W. (1996). *Adolescence: An introduction* (6th ed.). Madison, WI: Brown & Benchmark.

Savage, R. C. (2009). The developing brain after TBI: Predicting long-term deficits and services for children, adolescents, and young adults. *International Brain Injury Association*, Issue 04. Retrieved from http://www.internationalbrain.org/?q=node/112

Scheffler, A. (1997). *Let sleeping dogs lie and other proverbs from around the world.* Hauppauge, NY: Barron's.

Schickedanz, J. A., Schickedanz, D. I., Forsyth, P. D., & Forsyth, G. A. (2001). *Understanding children and adolescents* (4th ed.). Boston, MA: Allyn & Bacon.

Scott, C. M. (1988). A perspective on the evaluation of school children's narratives. *Language, Speech, and Hearing Services in Schools, 19*, 67–82.

Scott, C. (2004). Syntactic ability in children and adolescents with language and learning disabilities. In R. A. Berman (Ed.), *Language development across childhood and adolescence* (pp. 111–134). Philadelphia, PA: John Benjamins.

Scott, C. M. (2009). A case for the sentence in reading comprehension. *Language, Speech, and Hearing Services in Schools, 40*, 184–191.

Scott, C. (2010). Assessing expository texts produced by school-age children and adolescents. In M. A. Nippold & C. M. Scott (Eds.), *Expository discourse in children, adolescents, and adults: Development and disorders* (pp. 191–213). New York, NY: Psychology Press/Taylor & Francis.

Scott, C. M., & Nelson, N. W. (2009). Sentence combining: Assessment and intervention applications. *Perspectives on Language Learning and Education, 16*(1), 14–20.

Scott, C. M., & Windsor, J. (2000). General language performance measures in spoken and written narrative and expository discourse in school-age children with language learning disabilities. *Journal of Speech, Language, and Hearing Research, 43*, 324–339.

Searls, D. (Ed.). (2009). *The Journal, 1837–1861, Henry David Thoreau, Feb. 23, 1860 entry.* New York, NY: New York Review of Books.

Selman, R. L., Beardslee, W., Schultz, L. H., Krupa, M., & Podorefsky, D. (1986). Assessing adolescent interpersonal negotiation strategies: Toward the integration of structural and functional models. *Developmental Psychology, 22*, 450–459.

Semel, E., Wiig, E. H., & Secord, W. A. (1995). *Clinical evaluation of language fundamentals* (3rd ed.). San Antonio, TX: Psychological Corporation.

Semel, E., Wiig, E. H., & Secord, W. A. (2013). *Clinical evaluation of language fundamentals* (5th ed.). San Antonio, TX: Psychological Corporation.

Shea, V., & Mesibov, G. B. (2005). Adolescents and adults with autism. In F. R. Volkmar, R. Paul, A. Klin, & D. Cohen (Eds.), *Handbook of autism and pervasive developmental disorders, Volume 1: Diagnosis, development, neurobiology, and behavior* (3rd ed., pp. 288–311). Hoboken, NJ: John Wiley.

Sigman, M., & McGovern, C. W. (2005). Improvement in cognitive and language skills from preschool to adolescence in autism. *Journal of Autism and Developmental Disorders, 35*(1), 15–23.

Smith, K. J. (1995). *The nature of mathematics* (7th ed.). Pacific Grove, CA: Brooks/Cole.

Smith, M. (1926). An investigation of the development of the sentence and the extent of vocabulary in young children. *University of Iowa Studies in Child Welfare, 3*(5).

Stein, N. L., & Glenn, C. G. (1979). An analysis of story comprehension in elementary school children. In R. O. Freedle (Ed.), *New directions in discourse processing* (Vol. 2, pp. 53–120). Norwood, NJ: Ablex.

Stewart, J. (1997). *African proverbs and wisdom.* Secaucus, NJ: Carol Publishing/Citadel Press.

Strong, C. J., Mayer, M., & Mayer, M. (1998). *The Strong Narrative Assessment Procedure (SNAP).* Eau Claire, WI: Thinking Publications.

Style, S. (1993). *Honey: From hive to honeypot.* San Francisco, CA: Chronicle Books.

Sullivan, W. L. (2008). *Oregon's greatest natural disasters.* Eugene, OR: Navillus Press.

Sumner, W. G. (1906). *Folkways: A study of the sociological importance of usages, manners, customs, mores, and morals.* Boston, MA: Ginn.

Sun, L. & Nippold, M. A. (2012). Narrative writing in children and adolescents: Examining the literate lexicon. *Language, Speech, and Hearing Services in Schools, 43,* 2–13.

Tager-Flusberg, H. (2004). Strategies for conducting research on language in autism. *Journal of Autism and Developmental Disorders, 34,* 75–80.

Tager-Flusberg, H., Paul, R., & Lord, C. (2005). Language and communication in autism. In F. R. Volkmar, R. Paul, A. Klin, & D. Cohen (Eds.), *Handbook of autism and pervasive developmental disorders, Volume 1: Diagnosis, development, neurobiology, and behavior* (3rd ed., pp. 335–364). Hoboken, NJ: John Wiley.

Taine, H. (1877). On the acquisition of language by children. *Mind, 2,* 252–259.

Teachers need to be healthy. (2009, March 22). *The Register-Guard,* Eugene, OR, p. A12.

Tekiela, S. (2001). *Birds of Oregon field guide.* Cambridge, MN: Adventure Publications.

Templin, M. (1957). Certain language skills in children. *University of Minnesota Institute of Child Welfare Monograph Series 26.* Minneapolis, MN: University of Minnesota Press.

Thankful Kids. (2009, November 26). *The Register-Guard,* Eugene, OR, pp. A1, A12.

Thomas, D. (1954). *A child's Christmas in Wales.* New York, NY: New Directions.

Thoreau, H. D. (2004). *Walden: A fully annotated edition.* New Haven, CT: Yale University Press.

Tomalin, B. (2003). *Culture smart! France.* Portland, OR: Graphic Arts Center.

Tomblin, J. B., & Nippold, M. A. (2014). Features of language impairment in the school years. In J. B. Tomblin & M. A. Nippold (Eds.), *Understanding individual differences in language development across the school years* (pp. 79–116). New York, NY: Psychology Press/Taylor & Francis.

Toulmin, S. E. (1958). *The uses of argument.* London, UK: Cambridge University Press.

Trantham, C. R., & Pedersen, J. K. (1976). *Normal language development: The key to diagnosis and therapy for language-disordered children.* Baltimore, MD: Williams & Wilkins.

Tyack, D., & Gottsleben, R. (1974). *Language sampling, analysis, and training: A handbook for teachers and clinicians.* Palo Alto, CA: Consulting Psychologists Press.

Ukrainetz, T. A., & Gillam, R. B. (2009). The expressive elaboration of imaginative narratives by children with specific language impairment. *Journal of Speech, Language, and Hearing Research, 52,* 883–898.

Verhoeven, L., Aparici, M., Cahana-Amitay, D., van Hell, J., Kriz, S., & Viguie-Simon, A. (2002). Clause packaging in writing and speech: A cross-linguistic developmental analysis. *Written Language and Literacy, 5*(2), 135–162.

Volden, J., Coolican, J., Garon, N., White, J., & Bryson, S. (2009). Pragmatic language in autism spectrum disorder: Relationships to measures of ability and disability. *Journal of Autism and Developmental Disorders, 39,* 388–393.

Walker, H. M., Schwarz, I. E., & Nippold, M. A. (1994). Social skills in school-age children and youth: Issues and best practices in assessment and intervention. *Topics in Language Disorders, 14*(3), 70–82.

Ward-Lonergan, J. (2010). Expository discourse in school-age children and adolescents with language disorders: Nature of the problem. In M. A. Nippold & C. M. Scott (Eds.), *Expository discourse in children, adolescents, and adults: Development and disorders* (pp. 155–189). New York, NY: Psychology Press/Taylor & Francis.

Ward-Lonergan, J. M., Liles, B. Z., & Anderson, A. M. (1999). Verbal retelling abilities in adolescents with and without language-learning disabilities for social studies lectures. *Journal of Learning Disabilities, 32*(3), 213–223.

Who said? Volume II: A knowledge cards deck of memorable quotes. (2003). Rohnert Park, CA: Pomegranate.

Wiig, E. H., & Semel, E. M. (1976). *Language disabilities in children and adolescents.* Columbus, OH: Merrill.

Wikipedia. (2009). *Tape recorder.* Retrieved from http://www.en.wikipedia.org/wiki/tape_recorder

Williams, F. C. (2000). *Irish proverbs: Traditional wit & wisdom.* New York, NY: Sterling.

Wilson, D. L. (2006). *Lincoln's sword: The presidency and the power of words.* New York, NY: Knopf.

Wilson, N., & Murphy, A. (2008). *Scotland.* Oakland, CA: Lonely Planet Publications.

Windsor, J., Scott, C. M., & Street, C. K. (2000). Verb and noun morphology in the spoken and written language of children with language learning disabilities. *Journal of Speech, Language, and Hearing Research, 43*, 1322–1336.

Wong, B., Butler, D., Ficzere, S., & Kuperis, S. (1996). Teaching low achievers and students with learning disabilities to plan, write, and revise opinion essays. *Journal of Learning Disabilities, 29*, 197–212.

Wood, J. R., Weinstein, E. A., & Parker, R. (1967). Children's interpersonal tactics. *Sociological Inquiry, 37*, 129–138.

Wright, M., & Walters, S. (1980). *The book of the cat.* New York, NY: Summit Books.

Index

Note: Page numbers in **bold** reference non-text material.

H